Substance Abuse - New Compounds and New Problems

Edited by Javier Navarro-Zaragoza

Published in London, United Kingdom

Substance Abuse - New Compounds and New Problems
http://dx.doi.org/10.5772/intechopen.1005953
Edited by Javier Navarro-Zaragoza

Contributors
A. Esra Ismen Gazioglu, Bilge Nuran Aydogdu, Cigdem Demir Celebi, Derya Eryigit, Elena Martínez Laorden, Fatima Martín Sánchez, Halime Yildirim Hos, Javier Navarro-Zaragoza, Josep M. Ramon-Torrell, Lucía Fernández-López, Maanda Ravhutendele, Matome M. Sekhotha, Neslihan Yaman, Onkgopotse O. Ntsoane, Pholoso V. Ngwana, Pilar Almela Rojo, Raviye Ozen Koca, Seher Merve Erus, Seyma Arslan, Thabang O.L. Sekhotha, Tuanthon Boonlue, Zulfikare Isik Solak Gormus

First published in London, United Kingdom, 2025 by IntechOpen
IntechOpen is the global imprint of INTECHOPEN LIMITED, registered in England and Wales, registration number: 11086078, 167-169 Great Portland Street, London, W1W 5PF, United Kingdom

For EU product safety concerns: IN TECH d.o.o., Prolaz Marije Krucifikse Kozulić 3, 51000 Rijeka, Croatia, info@intechopen.com or visit our website at intechopen.com.

British Library Cataloguing-in-Publication Data
A catalogue record for this book is available from the British Library

Substance Abuse - New Compounds and New Problems
Edited by Javier Navarro-Zaragoza
p. cm.
Print ISBN 978-0-85466-473-3
Online ISBN 978-0-85466-472-6
eBook (PDF) ISBN 978-0-85466-474-0

If disposing of this product, please recycle the paper responsibly.

Meet the editor

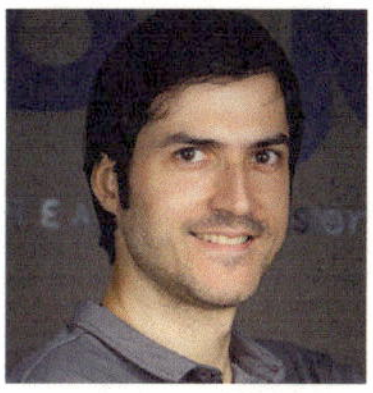

Dr. Navarro-Zaragoza is an Associate Professor in the Department of Pharmacology at the University of Murcia. He is the Head of the Department of Pharmacology at this university. He is the author of 35 scientific articles, five books, five book chapters, and three divulgation articles, as well as the author of 110 communications to national and international conferences. He was awarded his International Ph.D. from the University of Murcia in 2012, as well as degrees in Pharmacy (2007), Food Science and Technology (2013), and Human Nutrition and Dietetics (2009). He is the Head Director of the "Catedra Asgramur" at the University of Murcia, which researches severe asthma. He has been a scientific researcher at the University of Murcia since 2007, with stays at INSERM Neurocentre Magendie (Bordeaux, France) and Comenius University of Bratislava (Slovakia). He is a scientific researcher at the Murcian Institute for Biosanitary Research (IMIB-Arrixaca) involved in 7 national and four regional research projects with a funding of over 1. 2 million euros. He is a PI of 3 research contracts, and has two six-year research periods recognized by the CNEAI (2009-2014 and 2015-2020). He has directed five doctoral theses, and another four are currently in progress. He has also supervised 3 Master's Theses (TFM) and 31 Bachelor's Theses (TFG). He is a member of 11 scientific committees and has organized five scientific congresses. Additionally, he has served as chief in four study courses at the University of Murcia.

Contents

Preface

This Edited Volume is a compilation of peer-reviewed and relevant research chapters on advances in the field of substance abuse. We have included new compounds and new problems arising from their use. The book features academic contributions from several esteemed authors and has been edited and reviewed by a team of experts in the field of substance abuse. Each contribution is presented as a separate chapter, complete in itself, yet directly related to the book's themes and objectives.

The book consists of chapters that address different issues related to addiction, such as methamphetamine use and abuse, nicotine devices, adolescents and social media use, but also programmes to prevent addiction to tobacco and other drugs, or problems associated with drug use that affect different systems.

The target audience is academics and specialists in the field.

IntechOpen

Chapter 1

The Contemporary Addiction: Social Media Use and Its Impact on Well-Being

Lucía Fernández-López, Elena Martínez Laorden, Fatima Martín Sánchez, Pilar Almela Rojo and Javier Navarro-Zaragoza

Abstract

Social media are digital platforms that allow users to create, share, and view media content, as well as interact with each other through the internet. They facilitate communication, socialization, and the dissemination of information on a global scale. Its use presents many advantages. In addition to the fact that they provide entertainment, social media also facilitate instant communication and help with the dissemination of information in real time. Furthermore, from a business perspective, the visibility of brands is enhanced. Finally, they can also be used for educational and pedagogical purposes. Despite all these benefits, the use of social media also has a negative side. From a health perspective, social media can have negative effects on physical and mental health and can even lead to addiction. Social media addiction has been also found to be associated with numerous issues, including emotional, relational, health, and performance-related problems. Thus, this chapter aims to review the effect of social media use on the health of users.

Keywords: social media, internet, addiction, mental health, young people

1. Introduction

The presence of digital reality has accompanied people's daily lives for at least two decades, significantly impacting them [1, 2]. Nothing has made a greater impact in the way information is delivered to the average citizen in the past 30 years than the Internet. The Internet has transformed the way we research topics, explore new ideas, and communicate with one another. It has the potential to bring us closer—not only to the people we know but also to our colleagues and others we have never met except online [3].

As early as the 1990s, Internet addiction was studied by the American psychiatrist Ivan Goldberg, who coined the term Internet Addiction (1996), using the gambling disorder model as a reference to describe the addiction of spending excessive time on the computer browsing the web. This phenomenon was also equated with substance addiction [4] and later with impulse control disorder [5]. By the mid-1990s, excessive Internet use was classified as Internet Addiction Disorder [6], which is described as "a particular type of compulsive-impulsive disorder that manifests with symptoms such as an irresistible urge to connect to the web".

However, this broad term has evolved and now encompasses many types of addiction-related issues associated with generalized Internet addiction and a range of specific addictive Internet uses, including online gambling, online gaming, social networks, and cybersex, among others.

Access to the Internet is now very easy; you can connect anywhere with any type of device, whether it be a PC, a smartphone, or a tablet, 24 hours a day. In addition to that the rapid proliferation of Internet-based social media and the ways of interpersonal communication have drastically changed [7, 8]. Nowadays, young people do everything through digital technology, from chatting and shopping online to sharing photos and videos, with social media platforms at the top of the list for those who spend time online. In fact, as of October 2024, there were 5.52 billion internet users worldwide, representing 67.5% of the global population. Among them, 5.22 billion people (63.8% of the world's population) actively used social media. This indicates that most internet users also engage with social networking platforms [9].

2. Social media

Social networking is one of the most popular digital activities worldwide. Social media are digital platforms that allow users to create, share, and consume content, as well as interact with each other over the internet. They facilitate communication, socialization, and the dissemination of information on a global scale [10].

Social media enable communication between people through messages, comments, "likes," etc., in addition to sharing content, such as photos, videos, texts, and links. They facilitate relationships between individuals, businesses, and institutions regardless of geographical location, enabling a globalized connection. They also provide the possibility of creating "communities," which consist of groups of people with common interests, and they can adapt to users' interests and preferences, personalizing the experience.

The use of social media presents many advantages. In addition to providing opportunities to build and enhance friendships, receive social support, reduce feelings of isolation, social media facilitate instant communication and help with the dissemination of information in real time. Furthermore, from a business perspective, it enhances the visibility of brands and businesses and can also be used for educational and teaching purposes [11–13].

These platforms include Facebook, Instagram, Twitter, YikYak, WhatsApp, Snapchat, TikTok, WeChat, and others. These different types of social media vary depending on the user's main objective when connecting. Some are used for socializing and sharing diverse content (e.g., Facebook, Instagram, and Twitter/X), others focus on multimedia content, such as images and videos (e.g., TikTok, YouTube, and Pinterest). There are also professional/work-related platforms that promote professional connections and job opportunities (e.g., LinkedIn), and messaging platforms that allow direct communication between users (e.g., WhatsApp, Telegram).

2.1 Social media in numbers

Social media usage is one of the most popular online activities and it is no surprise that social networking penetration across all regions is constantly increasing. In 2024, over 5 billion people were using social media worldwide, a number projected to increase to over 6 billion in 2028 [14].

When Facebook launched in 2004, it changed the way people connect. Apps such as Messenger, Instagram, and WhatsApp further empowered billions around the world. In its launch year, Facebook reached 1 million users. By 2010, 500 million people were active on the platform, and by 2012, the number had grown to 1 billion. In 2017, Facebook reached 2 billion monthly users, while WhatsApp had 1 billion daily users. The following year, in 2018, Instagram reached 1 billion monthly users, and in 2021 WhatsApp amassing approximately 6 billion downloads. By 2023, Facebook had 2 billion daily active users [15]. As of April 2024, Facebook, YouTube, Instagram, and WhatsApp remain the most popular social networks worldwide, each surpassing 1 billion monthly active users [16].

The manner of accessing these platforms varies; however, it is primarily done through mobile phones. As of July 2021, it was found that 98.5% of active users accessed their Facebook account from mobile devices. In fact, almost 81.8% of Facebook audiences worldwide access the platform only via mobile phone [17].

In terms of the time spent, on average, internet users spend 151 minutes per day on social media and messaging apps, an increase of 40 minutes since 2015. On average, internet users in Latin America had the highest average time spent per day on social media [14].

As the data show, the use of social media is an activity with a very high consumption rate, and it tends to increase over time.

2.2 Social media during adolescence

Adolescence is a stage marked by significant emotional, social, and cognitive development. In this context, social media has become a fundamental means of interaction and self-expression [18]. Platforms such as Instagram, TikTok, Snapchat, and, to a lesser extent, Facebook, are used daily by millions of teenagers around the world, and this growing prevalence of social media use has sparked concerns about its potential effects on adolescents' health and well-being [11].

The Health Behavior in School-aged Children (HBSC) study, which surveyed nearly 280,000 adolescents across 44 countries in 2022, found that 11% of adolescents exhibit problematic social media behavior, with higher rates among girls (13%) than boys (9%). Besides, over a third (36%) stay in constant online contact with friends, particularly 15-year-old girls (44%) [19].

This use shows both the advantages and disadvantages. Social media enable adolescents to stay in touch with friends, meet new people, and strengthen interpersonal bonds. Moreover, these platforms offer a space for sharing interests, thoughts, or emotions, contributing to identity development, and, in some cases, they can serve as a source of peer support in the face of personal challenges. Moreover, on other side, they facilitate access to educational content, news, and cultural resources.

However, social media also show a negative side in adolescence stage. Constant exposure to idealized images can generate feelings of inadequacy, anxiety, or depression [20]. Adolescents may be vulnerable to sharing personal information without fully understanding the associated risks, which could affect their privacy or even their security [21]. Moreover, with the explosion of a variety of platforms over the last decade, social media have emerged as the most common vehicles for cyberbullying victimization and perpetration, with serious psychological consequences [22, 23].

The excessive use may lead to dependence, negatively impacting areas, such as academic performance and sleep quality. Problematic social media use is defined by addiction-like symptoms, including an inability to control usage, withdrawal symptoms, neglect of other activities, and negative life consequences. Research links it to poor mental and social well-being, substance use, sleep issues, and lower academic performance [11, 24]. Dr. Hans Henri P. Kluge, WHO Regional Director for Europe, emphasizes the need for better digital literacy education and immediate action to address the issue. Some governments are considering restrictions or bans on social media for younger children to mitigate its negative effects, which can include depression, bullying, anxiety, and academic struggles [25].

2.3 Negative consequences in general population

Social media have become a necessity for everyone; it is almost impossible to do without it. Teenagers constantly update their personal profiles and check their homepages, tapping on social media app icons on their smartphones without respecting usage limits [26]. However, the use of social media has an important negative side.

The ease of sharing information can lead to the spread of false information or "fake news". Using social media for news consumption is a double-edged sword. On one hand, its low cost, easy accessibility, and rapid information dissemination encourage people to turn to social media for news. On the other hand, it facilitates the widespread distribution of "fake news," meaning low-quality information that intentionally contains false content. The extensive spread of such content can have highly negative effects on both individuals and society [27].

Currently, there is growing concern about privacy and data security risks, especially among minors. Teenagers disclose a variety of personal information on social media platforms, which are specifically designed to promote sharing and network growth. However, most teens do not opt for a completely public presence online. Instead, they implement various strategies to limit and carefully manage their profiles [21].

Previous researches have demonstrated that Millennials have a strong desire to live publicly, willingly sharing information that was once considered private online. However, despite this openness, findings indicate that they still expect a certain level of privacy within their networks and prefer to keep their audiences separate, expressing strong opposition to being compelled to share their content with unintended viewers [28].

Another negative consequence of using social media is that it affects academic performance. Previous studies have found that the amount of time one spends using social media is negatively correlated with their academic performance [24, 29–31]. Specifically, Sampasa-Kanyinga et al. [31] found that spending 2 hours or less per day on social media use was positively linked to higher levels of school connectedness among high school students. In contrast, social media use exceeding 2 hours per day was negatively associated with school connectedness and academic performance. Additionally, the study found that the connection between social media use and school connectedness varied significantly by age, with stronger effects observed in older students. Gender did not play a significant role in moderating these relationships [31].

2.3.1 Negative health consequences

From a health perspective, social media can have negative effects on mental and physical health.

Inactivity, long sedentary time, and lack of sleep may impact young individual's physical and mental well-being. Too many hours hunched over a screen can lead to muscle pain, such as neck and shoulder pain, eye irritation, and difficulty focusing. Additionally, losing valuable sleep can have negative consequences in user's lives, such as fatigue, depression, obsessive-compulsive disorders, substance abuse, and poor academic performance. These health disorders can be influenced by various factors, including screen size, the number of text messages sent, and the hours spent each day [32–34].

The widespread availability of social media platforms and the easy access to the Internet may lead to the compulsive and excessive use of social media that it interferes with other aspects of daily life [35, 36]. This excessive use has even been associated with disordered eating and poorer body image outcomes [20].

Different terms have been used to refer to this behavior, such as problematic social media use or social media addiction [37], but social networking sites addiction has not yet been recognized as a legitimate disorder. However, recent research has indicated that the use of social media could become problematic and be characterized by addictive-type symptoms [38].

For people who develop this disorder, a type of social anxiety develops. The strong desire to stay connected with the activities of others and the fear of being excluded from events, experiences, or social contexts cause anxiety and a high level of stress in young people. The compulsive need to stay connected becomes so essential that it is impossible to do without it [39, 40].

Several studies have linked excessive social media use to lower psychological well-being [41]. Studies have also linked social media addiction to numerous issues, including emotional, relational, health, and performance-related problems [24]. Some studies suggest problematic social media use may lead to psychological distress and reduced well-being, while others argue it is actually a result of issues, such as depression, loneliness, or poor social health [42–44].

Since Facebook is still the most popular social network sites with more than 2 billion monthly users, most studies are done using Facebook. Research has found a link between problematic Facebook use and mental health issues, such as anxiety, depression, and loneliness. Users with depression may turn to Facebook to manage their mood [45], while socially anxious individuals might use it to compensate for low self-esteem and poor offline communication skills [46]. Although social media can offer short-term relief and a sense of support, it often does not lead to improved real-life social abilities. In some cases, it even serves as an escape from real-life problems, which may worsen symptoms, such as depression and suicidal thoughts [47]. Overall, problematic Facebook use is connected to several negative mental health outcomes [42].

Instagram has risen in popularity and recently reached a milestone of 1 billion monthly active users, and the majority of studies examine the relationship between Instagram use and indicators of body image and disordered eating. Researchers found strong evidence that links Instagram use with negative outcomes related to social comparison, body image dissatisfaction, and disordered eating behaviors [48–50], but the relationship between Instagram use and factors such as self-esteem, stress, and substance use, remains unclear due to limited or inconsistent findings [18]. There is a need for more longitudinal and experimental studies to better understand causal relationships and underlying psychological mechanisms.

YouTube is one of the most visited web platforms in the world. It allows anyone to create, share, and consume videos worldwide, and its influence extends across education, culture, entertainment, and even mental health. In this regard, a review of 32 empirical and theoretical studies examining how YouTube usage influences mental health found that while YouTube offers beneficial resources for mental health support, its impact is nuanced. Frequent YouTube users, especially those below 29 years old, exhibit higher levels of loneliness, anxiety, and depression, and this is notably prevalent among individuals who regularly watch content about other people's lives [51].

Different studies have investigated how depression, bipolar disorder, and general mental health are portrayed on YouTube and the implications of these portrayals on public perceptions, stigma, and mental health literacy [52, 53]. The authors emphasize that YouTube serves as a significant platform for disseminating information about mental health. However, the predominance of content created by non-professionals highlights the need for more balanced and accurate narratives that can improve mental health literacy and reduce stigma [53]. Additionally, they stress the powerful role of personal storytelling in engaging audiences on mental health topics, while also pointing to the need for guidance in assessing the quality and reliability of such content [52]. Overall, it highlighted the importance of strategic interventions to strengthen YouTube's role in promoting mental well-being.

Another one of the most popular and most recent social networks is TikTok. The international version of TikTok was launched in September 2017, and by the end of 2024, TikTok had more than 1840 million monthly active users worldwide.

A systematic review and content analysis of how TikTok is used in the context of public and youth mental health examined existing literature and analyzed TikTok content to assess the platform's role in disseminating mental health information, shaping perceptions, and influencing behaviors among young users [54]. The study found that TikTok has emerged as a significant platform where youth actively engage with mental health topics, both through content creation and consumption. Videos often address issues, such as anxiety, depression, self-care, and therapy, frequently using humor, personal storytelling, or trends to communicate messages [54].

O'Donnell et al. [55] examined how TikTok's #EduTok campaign disseminates health-related content and engages audiences. By analyzing 400 videos, the researchers aimed to understand the effectiveness of educational and motivational health messages on the platform. The study suggests that while TikTok can be an effective platform for health education, the content often prioritizes engagement over informative value. Health professionals and educators are encouraged to collaborate with influencers to create content that combines personal storytelling with evidence-based information, ensuring that messages are both relatable and actionable. This approach could enhance the credibility and effectiveness of health communication on social media platforms [55].

While TikTok offers opportunities for raising awareness and reducing stigma, studies also highlight concerns regarding the accuracy of information, potential for misinformation, and the platform's impact on vulnerable populations. The authors call for increased collaboration between mental health professionals and content creators, as well as the development of guidelines to ensure safe and effective communication on the platform [54, 56].

2.4 Social media and drug consumption

Due to the widespread and global use of social media, recent research has explored how these platforms can be used to identify or detect patterns of substance use, as well as how social media influence drug consumption, whether it promotes or reduces it.

Studies have examined how feedback on social media influences individuals who disclose drug consumption online. Authors analyzed user's posts related to drug use and examined the type and tone of feedback received—such as supportive, neutral, or critical responses. The research found that feedback plays a significant role in shaping future behavior and content shared by users. Specifically, supportive feedback was more likely to encourage further disclosure and engagement, while critical or negative feedback could lead to reduced posting or changes in how individuals talked about their drug use. The paper suggests that understanding these interactions can help design more effective online interventions and support systems for people at risk of substance abuse [57].

Other articles have explored how social media big data can be used to enhance research on drug abuse and addiction [58–61]. Authors have argued that traditional methods such as surveys and clinical studies are limited in scale and timeliness. In contrast, social media platforms provide real-time, large-scale, and naturally occurring data that reflect people's behaviors, emotions, and social interactions [58].

The authors have discussed the potential of data from platforms such as Twitter, Reddit, and Facebook to uncover trends in drug use, identify at-risk populations, and inform public health interventions. They have highlighted the use of machine learning, natural language processing (NLP), and data mining techniques to analyze this unstructured data [58–61].

Castillo-Toledo et al. [62] analyzed Twitter data to explore how cocaine is discussed online, focusing on public perceptions, patterns of use, and geographical differences. The authors conducted a cross-sectional analysis of tweets containing cocaine-related keywords to identify trends and regional variations in discourse, and they concluded that Twitter can serve as a valuable tool for real-time drug trend surveillance, helping inform public health efforts [62].

A systematic review examined a range of studies that analyze user-generated content on platforms such as Twitter, Instagram, and Reddit to monitor drug-related behaviors and trends [59]. The review found that social media can serve as a valuable tool for early detection of emerging drug use patterns, geographic hotspots, and public sentiment around substances. Various computational techniques, including natural language processing and image analysis, were used in the studies reviewed [59, 60].

Other findings suggest that social media data can reveal meaningful patterns in how individuals transition from one drug to another, which may be useful for early intervention and prevention strategies [60].

Despite the opportunities, the authors also address several challenges, including privacy concerns, ethical considerations, and data quality. They caution about the limitations of interpreting social media content, such as the presence of irony, sarcasm, and the lack of representativeness in the data. They call for interdisciplinary collaboration and the development of standardized frameworks to responsibly and effectively use social media data for addiction research [58–62].

3. Conclusions

The use of social media constitutes a powerful tool that, when managed appropriately, can provide significant benefits for both personal and social development, including opportunities for communication, learning, self-expression, and the creation of supportive communities. Nevertheless, a growing body of research highlights that excessive or unregulated engagement with these platforms is associated with a variety of health-related issues. This correlation appears to be particularly pronounced among the most vulnerable segments of the population—adolescents—who are in a critical stage of cognitive, emotional, and social development. The negative consequences most frequently reported include increased levels of anxiety, depression, sleep disturbances, and diminished self-esteem, often linked to mechanisms such as social comparison, cyberbullying, or the constant exposure to unrealistic standards of success and beauty. For these reasons, it is essential to encourage a more critical and responsible use of social media, emphasizing the development of digital literacy skills from an early age. This process requires the active involvement not only of individuals but also of families, educators, and institutions, who must work together to create environments that foster healthy online habits, promote resilience, and mitigate potential risks while still enabling young people to take advantage of the positive aspects that these technologies can offer.

Conflict of interest

The authors declare no conflict of interest.

Author details

Lucía Fernández-López, Elena Martínez Laorden, Fatima Martín Sánchez, Pilar Almela Rojo and Javier Navarro-Zaragoza*
Department of Pharmacology, University of Murcia, Murcia, Spain

*Address all correspondence to: jnavarrozaragoza@um.es

References

[1] Giedd JN. The digital revolution and adolescent brain evolution. Journal of Adolescent Health. 2012;**51**(2):101-105. DOI: 10.1016/j.jadohealth.2012.06.002

[2] King D, Delfabbro P. Internet Gaming Disorder: Theory, Assessment, Treatment, and Prevention. Academic Press; 2018. p. 294. RRP:117.95;153.93 (e-book). ISBN 978012819241

[3] Barak A, Grohol JM. Current and future trends in internet-supported mental health interventions. Journal of Technology in Human Services. 2011;**29**(3):155-196

[4] Young K. Psychology of computer use: XL. Addictive use of the internet: A case that breaks the stereotype. Psychological Reports. 1996;**79**(3):899-902. DOI: 10.2466/pr0.1996.79.3.899

[5] Young K, Rogers RC. The relationship between depression and internet addiction. CyberPsychology and Behavior. 1998;**1**(1):25-28. DOI: 10.1089/cpb.1998.1.25

[6] Block JJ. Issues for DSM-V: Internet addiction. American Journal of Psychiatry. 2008;**165**(3):306-307

[7] Smith A, Anderson M. Social media use in 2018. Washington, DC, USA: Pew Research Center; 2018. Available from: http://www.pewinternet.org/2018/03/01/social-media-use-in-2018/ [Accessed: May 23, 2025]

[8] Stone CB, Wang Q. From conversations to digital communication: The mnemonic consequences of consuming and sharing information via social media. Topics in Cognitive Science. 2018;**2018**:1-20. DOI: 10.1111/tops.12369

[9] Petrosyan A. Worldwide Digital Population 2025. 2025. Available from: https://www.statista.com/statistics/617136/digital-population-worldwide/ [Accessed: May 23, 2025]

[10] Bayer JB, Triệu P, Ellison NB. Social media elements, ecologies, and effects. Annual Review of Psychology. 2020;**71**(1):471-497

[11] Boniel-Nissim M, van den Eijnden RJ, Furstova J, Marino C, Lahti H, Inchley J, et al. International perspectives on social media use among adolescents: Implications for mental and social well-being and substance use. Computers in Human Behavior. 2022;**129**:107144

[12] Allen KA, Ryan T, Gray DL, McInerney DM, Waters L. Social media use and social connectedness in adolescents: The positives and the potential pitfalls. The Educational and Developmental Psychologist. 2014;**31**(1):18-31

[13] Clark JL, Algoe SB, Green MC. Social network sites and well-being: The role of social connection. Current Directions in Psychological Science. 2018;**27**(1):32-37

[14] Dixon SJ. Number of Global Social Network Users 2017-2028. 2025. Available from: https://www.statista.com/statistics/278414/number-of-worldwide-social-network-users/ [Accessed: May 23, 2025]

[15] Meta. (s.f.). Available from: https://about.meta.com/company-info/?utm_source=about.facebook.com&utm_medium=redirect [Accessed: May 23, 2025]

[16] Dixon SJ. Most Used Social Networks 2025, by Number of Users. 2025.

Available from: https://www.statista.com/statistics/272014/global-social-networks-ranked-by-number-of-users/ [Accessed: May 23, 2025]

[17] Dixon SJ. Countries with the Most Facebook Users 2024. 2024. Available from: https://www.statista.com/statistics/268136/top-15-countries-based-on-number-of-facebook-users/#:~:text=As%20of%20July%202021%2C%20it,amassing%20approximately%20six%20billion%20downloads [Accessed: May 23, 2025]

[18] Faelens L, Hoorelbeke K, Cambier R, Van Put J, Van de Putte E, De Raedt R, et al. The relationship between Instagram use and indicators of mental health: A systematic review. Computers in Human Behavior Reports. 2021;**4**:100121

[19] Boniel-Nissim M, Marino C, Galeotti T, Blinka L, Ozoliņa K, et al. A focus on adolescent social media use and gaming in Europe, central Asia and Canada. Health Behaviour in School-aged Children international report from the 2021/2022 survey. Volume 6. Copenhagen: WHO Regional Office for Europe; 2024. CC BY-NC-SA 3.0 IGO

[20] Holland G, Tiggemann M. A systematic review of the impact of the use of social networking sites on body image and disordered eating outcomes. Body Image. 2016;**17**:100-110

[21] Madden M, Lenhart A, Cortesi S, Gasser U, Duggan M, Smith A, et al. Teens, social media, and privacy. Pew Research Center. 2013;**21**(1055):2-86

[22] Giumetti GW, Kowalski RM. Cyberbullying via social media and well-being. Current Opinion in Psychology. 2022;**45**:101314

[23] Kowalski RM, Dillon E, Macbeth J, Franchi M, Bush M. Racial differences in cyberbullying from the perspective of victims and perpetrators. American journal of orthopsychiatry. 2020;**90**(5):644

[24] Hou Y, Xiong D, Jiang T, Song L, Wang Q. Social media addiction: Its impact, mediation, and intervention. Cyberpsychology: Journal of Psychosocial Research on Cyberspace. 2019;**13**(1):Article 4. DOI: 10.5817/CP2019-1-4

[25] Conroy G. Governments are banning kids from social media: Will that protect them from harm? Nature. 2024;**636**(8043):530-531

[26] Al Qudah DA, Al-Shboul B, Al-Sayyed R, Cristea AI. Investigating users' experience on social media ads: Perceptions of young users. Heliyon. 2020;**6**(7):e04378

[27] Shu K, Sliva A, Wang S, Tang J, Liu H. Fake news detection on social media: A data mining perspective. ACM SIGKDD explorations newsletter. 2017;**19**(1):22-36

[28] Abril PS, Levin A, Del Riego A. Blurred boundaries: Social media privacy and the twenty-first-century employee. American Business Law Journal. 2012;**49**:63

[29] Al-Menayes J. The relationship between mobile social media use and academic performance in university students. New Media and Mass Communication. 2014;**25**(2):23-29

[30] Al-Menayes JJ. Social media use, engagement and addiction as predictors of academic performance. International Journal of Psychological Studies. 2015;**7**(4):86-94

[31] Sampasa-Kanyinga H, Chaput JP, Hamilton HA. Social media use, school connectedness, and academic

performance among adolescents. The Journal of Primary Prevention. 2019;**40**:189-211

[32] Al-Samarraie H, Bello KA, Alzahrani AI, Smith AP, Emele C. Young users' social media addiction: Causes, consequences and preventions. Information Technology and People. 2022;**35**(7):2314-2343

[33] Christensen M, Bettencourt L, Kaye L, Moturu ST, Nguyen KT, Olgin JE, et al. Direct measurements of smartphone screen-time: Relationships with demographics and sleep. PLoS One. 2016;**11**(11):e0165331. DOI: 10.1371/journal.pone.0165331

[34] Mahapatra S. Smartphone addiction and associated consequences: Role of loneliness and self-regulation. Behaviour and Information Technology. 2019;**38**(8):833-844. DOI: 10.1080/0144929x.2018

[35] Griffiths MD. Internet addiction: Time to be taken seriously? Addiction Research. 2000;**8**:413-418. DOI: 10.3109/16066350009005587

[36] Griffiths MD. Facebook addiction: Concerns, criticism, and recommendations: A response to Andreassen and colleagues. Psychological Reports. 2012;**110**:518-520. DOI: 10.2466/01.07.18.PR0.110.2.518-520

[37] Błachnio A, Przepiórka A, Pantic I. Internet use, Facebook intrusion, and depression: Results of a cross-sectional study. European Psychiatry. 2015;**30**(6):681-684

[38] Griffiths MD, Kuss DJ, Demetrovics Z. Social networking addiction: An overview of preliminary findings. In Rosenberg KP, Curtiss Feder L, editors, Behavioral Addictions: Criteria, Evidence, and Treatment. London: Elsevier Inc.; 2014. p. 119-141. DOI: 10.1016/B978-0-12-407724-9.00006-9

[39] Braumüller B. Young adults' perceptions of the relevance of interaction on social online networks for sports activities. European Journal for Sport and Society. 2020;**17**(3):231-249. DOI: 10.1080/16138171.2020.1792072

[40] Caplan SE. Problematic internet use and psychosocial well-being: Development of a theory-based cognitive–behavioral measurement instrument. Computers in Human Behavior. 2002;**18**(5):553-575

[41] Huang C. Time spent on social network sites and psychological well-being: A meta-analysis. Cyberpsychology, Behavior, and Social Networking. 2017;**20**(6):346-354

[42] Marino C, Gini G, Vieno A, Spada MM. The associations between problematic Facebook use, psychological distress and well-being among adolescents and young adults: A systematic review and meta-analysis. Journal of Affective Disorders. 2018;**226**:274-281

[43] Schou Andreassen C, Pallesen S. Social network site addiction-an overview. Current Pharmaceutical Design. 2014;**20**(25):4053-4061

[44] Balci Ş, Gölcü A. Facebook addiction among university students in Turkey: Selçuk University example. Journal of Turkish Studies. 2013;**34**:255-278

[45] Hong FY, Huang DH, Lin HY, Chiu SL. Analysis of the psychological traits, Facebook usage, and Facebook addiction model of Taiwanese university students. Telematics and Informatics. 2014;**31**(4):597-606

[46] Bodroža B, Jovanović T. Validation of the new scale for measuring behaviors of Facebook users: Psycho-social aspects of Facebook use (PSAFU). Computers in Human Behavior. 2016;**54**:425-435

[47] Walburg V, Mialhes A, Moncla D. Does school-related burnout influence problematic Facebook use? Children and Youth Services Review. 2016;**61**:327-331

[48] Åberg E, Koivula A, Kukkonen I. A feminine burden of perfection? Appearance-related pressures on social networking sites. Telematics and Informatics. 2020;**46**:101319

[49] Fardouly J, Magson NR, Rapee RM, Johnco CJ, Oar EL. The use of social media by Australian preadolescents and its links with mental health. Journal of Clinical Psychology. 2020;**76**(7):1304-1326

[50] Wilksch SM, O'Shea A, Ho P, Byrne S, Wade TD. The relationship between social media use and disordered eating in young adolescents. International Journal of Eating Disorders. 2020;**53**(1):96-106

[51] Balcombe L, De Leo D. The impact of youtube on loneliness and mental health. In: Informatics. Vol. 10, No. 2. MDPI; 2023. p. 39. DOI: 10.3390/informatics10020039

[52] Oliphant T. User engagement with mental health videos on YouTube. Journal of the Canadian Health Libraries Association/Journal de l'Association des bibliothèques de la santé du Canada. 2013;**34**(3):153-158

[53] Devendorf A, Bender A, Rottenberg J. Depression presentations, stigma, and mental health literacy: A critical review and YouTube content analysis. Clinical Psychology Review. 2020;**78**:101843

[54] McCashin D, Murphy CM. Using TikTok for public and youth mental health–a systematic review and content analysis. Clinical Child Psychology and Psychiatry. 2023;**28**(1):279-306

[55] O'Donnell N, Jerin SI, Mu D. Using TikTok to educate, influence, or inspire? A content analysis of health-related EduTok videos. Journal of Health Communication. 2023;**28**(8):539-551

[56] Milton A, Ajmani L, DeVito MA, Chancellor S. "I see me here": Mental health content, community, and algorithmic curation on TikTok. In: Proceedings of the 2023 CHI Conference on Human Factors in Computing Systems. 2023. pp. 1-17

[57] Jangra H, Shah R, Kumaraguru P. Effect of feedback on drug consumption disclosures on social media. In: Proceedings of the International AAAI Conference on Web and Social Media. Vol. 17. 2023. pp. 435-446

[58] Kim SJ, Marsch LA, Hancock JT, Das AK. Scaling up research on drug abuse and addiction through social media big data. Journal of Medical Internet Research. 2017;**19**(10):e353

[59] Kazemi DM, Borsari B, Levine MJ, Dooley B. Systematic review of surveillance by social media platforms for illicit drug use. Journal of Public Health. 2017;**39**(4):763-776

[60] Yuan Y, Kasson E, Taylor J, Cavazos-Rehg P, De Choudhury M, Aledavood T. Examining the gateway hypothesis and mapping substance use pathways on social media: Machine learning approach. JMIR Formative Research. 2024;**8**:e54433

[61] Fisher A, Young MM, Payer D, Pacheco K, Dubeau C, Mago V. Automating detection of drug-related harms on social media: Machine learning framework. Journal of Medical Internet Research. 2023;**25**:e43630

[62] Castillo-Toledo C, Fraile-Martínez O, Donat-Vargas C, Lara-Abelenda FJ, Ortega MA, Garcia-Montero C, et al. Insights from the Twittersphere: A cross-sectional study of public perceptions, usage patterns, and geographical differences of tweets discussing cocaine. Frontiers in Psychiatry. 2024;**15**:1282026

Chapter 2

A School-Based Life Skills Program for Preventing Adolescent Substance Use: Insights from Türkiye

A. Esra Ismen Gazioglu, Seher Merve Erus, Cigdem Demir Celebi, Neslihan Yaman, Derya Eryigit, Bilge Nuran Aydogdu, Halime Yildirim Hos and Seyma Arslan

Abstract

This chapter introduces a school-based life skills education program and its effectiveness among Turkish adolescents. "Green Crescent Life Skills Program (GCLS)" was developed and revised according to the results of its pilot implementation. A 2 × 3 mixed factorial design with pre-post and follow-up measurements was used to test the effectiveness of the program. A total of 388 seventh-grade students participated in the intervention and control groups. After the descriptive analysis and assumption checks, two-way ANOVAs were employed to analyze the significant interaction effects across dependent variables. Results of the study showed that the program was effective in improving life skills and self-efficacy for protecting substance use, and the significant effects were found to be stable across the follow-up measurements. The results showed that a GCLS program was effective in promoting life skills that targeted preventing tobacco, alcohol, and substance use in Turkish seventh-grade students. In the present study, an easily accessible, school-based prevention program has been developed, aiming to promote an alcohol, tobacco, and drug-free lifestyle among adolescents within the scope of substance use prevention.

Keywords: substance use prevention, life skills, school-based prevention program, prevention in Türkiye, green crescent life skills program

1. Introduction

School-based programs serve as essential interventions within educational settings, designed to enhance students' social and emotional skills while mitigating psychological and social risks to their mental well-being [1, 2]. By reaching a large and diverse student population through well-structured and cost-effective plans, these programs play a vital role in preventive and therapeutic strategies for children and adolescents [3]. Schools, as important environments for socialization, are critical settings for promoting mental health, as many children and adolescents face barriers to accessing psychological services due to social, emotional, and behavioral challenges in their daily lives [4]. Within these settings, schools can identify at-risk students, enhance well-being, and enable the provision of early interventions for effectively addressing mental health concerns [5]. The widespread attendance of children and adolescents at schools has led to an increasing emphasis on school-based prevention and early intervention programs. School-based programs are designed to foster overall mental health and commonly focus on preventing and intervening in challenges such as depression and anxiety, as well as tobacco, substance, and internet addiction [6–8]. Thus, integrating such evidence-based strategies into school settings can significantly contribute to reducing substance use and enhancing mental health among adolescents.

School-based drug prevention (SBDP) programs are especially popular, with evidence indicating that their benefits are twice the cost [9]. SBDP programs aimed at preventing tobacco, alcohol, and substance use include five different types of interventions, each based on a different theoretical orientation. These are [10]: (1) Information-only curricula that provide information to oppose tobacco [alcohol, and substance] use (e.g., [11–13]), (2) Social competence curricula that aim to help adolescents refuse offers to tobacco [alcohol, and substance] use by enhancing their general social competence through social learning processes or life skills (e.g., [13, 14]), (3) Social influence curricula that aim to overcome social pressures promoting tobacco use by providing skills to adolescents (also called social skills interventions) (e.g., [15, 16]), (4) Combined social competence and social influences curricula, (5) Multimodal programs that combine curricular approaches with broader initiatives both within and outside the school, including programs for parents, schools, communities, and other initiatives (e.g., [17, 18]). A previous study comparatively examining the effectiveness of different types of SBDP programs showed that programs that develop individual social skills are the most effective form of school-based intervention for the prevention of early substance use and should be selected when planning community interventions against substance use [7]. Adolescence is a critical period for the onset of substance use [19, 20]. Therefore, intervention programs that aim to prevent the use of substances among adolescents are considered to be of crucial importance in Western and non-Western contexts.

Research on the age of onset of substance use in Türkiye aligns with findings from Western societies, identifying 15 years as a critical age (e.g., [21]). However, more current studies indicate an earlier initiation of substance use [22, 23]. Alcohol is the most commonly used substance among Turkish adolescents [24–26], while tobacco and alcohol use are less prevalent compared to European countries. Illicit substance use in Türkiye remains below the global average, but there has been an increase in substance use over recent years. Despite lower substance use prevalence than in Western societies, these trends highlight the need for prevention and intervention programs for adolescents in Türkiye [27–30]. Evidence-based interventions represent a critical yet underexplored component of substance prevention efforts in Türkiye. Interventions aimed at preventing substance use in Türkiye are generally of an information-only type [31–33]. The Training Program on Addiction Prevention of Türkiye (TPAP) is one of the evidence-based programs implemented at the national level in Türkiye [34]. TPAP is the only type of intervention that focuses on multiple age groups, ranging from childhood to adulthood. The Program on Addiction Intervention in Schools (AIS) is another evidence-based program focused on children and adolescents who have experimented with or engaged in substance use but have not yet developed an addiction [35]. Despite the limited number of life skills-based prevention programs aimed at reducing substance use among Turkish adolescents [36, 37], only one study assessing the effectiveness of such programs has been reported [38]. Current empirical evidence regarding the effectiveness of these programs remains limited and inconsistent. In this context, we concluded that there is a critical need for programs focused on the development of social competencies as an alternative to information-based prevention programs in Türkiye. To address this need, we developed the Green Crescent Life Skills (GCLS) program. Considering that early intervention before the critical age of 15 is crucial for preventing substance use, we selected seventh-grade students as our target group. The GCLS program seeks to empower adolescents with the skills and knowledge to prevent substance use. During the development of the GCLS program, the initial phase involved identifying the key life skills to be prioritized. According to WHO, life skills include communication and interpersonal skills, decision-making and critical thinking competencies, coping and self-management strategies, as well as the use of alcohol, tobacco, and other substances [5]. The content of the GCLS program has been designed by considering the developmental characteristics of the target group, the life skills recommended by WHO for substance use prevention, and various evidence-based life skills programs [39–43]. In this regard, the GCLS program has been structured based on the areas of self-awareness and body image, coping with negative emotions, and peer relationships. These three main areas of the program were addressed through in-class experiential activities. After the activities were completed, questions on the implementation and personalization processes were asked first, followed by action ideas and daily life adaptation questions to get students thinking about the program area addressed. Previous research has demonstrated that school-based life skills programs have beneficial effects on risk factors associated with adolescent substance use [39, 44]. However, the majority of school-based prevention programs targeting substance use in Türkiye are usually information-based prevention programs rather than incorporating a comprehensive life skills approach. These knowledge-based programs have suffered from a lack of methodological rigor. The present study addresses this gap by conducting a pretest-posttest control group design to evaluate the effectiveness of a school-based life skills program in enhancing students' life skills. This study aims to address these gaps and contribute to the global understanding of life skills-based prevention programs, particularly in non-Western contexts like Türkiye. Based on previous research, we hypothesized that firstly, the GCLS program has positive effects on self-awareness and body image, coping with negative emotions, thinking skills, and peer relationships life skills in Turkish adolescents; secondly, the program positively affects the self-efficacy skills in avoiding substance use; and thirdly, the program positively affects the rejection of alcohol, tobacco, and other substances.

2. Method

2.1 Design

The design of this study was a 2 × 3 (pretest-posttest follow-up with a control group) factorial design. To ensure representativeness of schools across Türkiye, intervention schools were selected from nine different cities within the scope of the Nomenclature of Territorial Units for Statistics Level 1 (NUTS-1). From each of the nine cities, one school was selected for the intervention group and one for the control group. One class from each selected school was randomly assigned to either the intervention or control group. Additionally, for the control group, schools with characteristics similar to those of the intervention schools (e.g., school size and students' demographics) were selected in each city.

The intervention and control groups consisted of the schools where the trained GCLS program facilitators work as school psychological counselors in each city. The GCLS program was implemented in the intervention groups (IG), and the control groups (CG) were placed on the waiting list. Moreover, pretest, posttest, and follow-up measurements were conducted in both groups concurrently. The measurements for the pretest of the study were conducted in both groups approximately 1 week before the implementation of the program. Posttest measurements were taken immediately following the completion of the program (approximately 8 weeks after the pretest), and follow-up measurements were obtained approximately 6 weeks after the posttest (see **Table 1**). The independent variable in this study was the GCLS program, while the dependent variables included students' life skills, self-efficacy in avoiding substance use, and refusal skills for alcohol, tobacco, and other substances.

2.2 Study group

The study group comprised 449 seventh-grade students, including 206 in the control group and 243 in the intervention group. **Table 1** provides an overview of

Region	**City**	**Seventh grade**	
		Intervention (n)	**Control (n)**
Istanbul	İstanbul	23	14
West Marmara Tekirdağ, Edirne, Kırklareli, Balıkesir, Çanakkale	Çanakkale	33	22
Ege İzmir, Aydın, Denizli,Muğla, Manisa, Afyonkarahisar, Kütahya, Uşak	İzmir	30	30
East Marmara Bursa, Eskişehir, Bilecik, Kocaeli, Sakarya, Düzce, Bolu, Yalova	Eskişehir	24	18
Western Anatolia Ankara, Konya, Karaman	Ankara	32	25
Mediterranean Antalya, Isparta, Burdur, Adana, Mersin, Osmaniye Kahramanmaraş, Hatay	Mersin	18	16
Eastern Black Sea Trabzon, Ordu, Giresun, Rize, Artvin, Gümüşhane	Rize	25	24
Northeast Anatolia Erzurum, Erzincan, Ağrı Ardahan Bayburt, Kars, Iğdır	Erzurum	25	28
Southeast Anatolia Gaziantep, Şanlıurfa, Siirt Mardin, Kilis, Diyarbakır, Batman, Şırnak, Adıyaman	Gaziantep	33	29
Total		243	206

Table 1.
GCLS program study group distribution.

the NUTS-1 level cities where the GCLS program was implemented, along with the number of students who participated in the intervention process in each city.

In the intervention group, 45.2% (n = 102) of the students were female and 54.8% (n = 132) were male. The majority of students (57.4%, n = 139) were 12 years old, while 36% (n = 87) were 13 years old. In the control group, 54.7% (n = 111) of the students were female and 45.3% (n = 92) were male. Similarly, 58.7% (n = 121) were 12 years old, and 32% (n = 66) were 13 years old.

Considering the income level, 29% (n = 58) of the intervention group were in the range of 1501–2500 TL and 27.5% (n = 55) were in the range of 2501–5000 TL. In the control group, 34.3% (n = 62) were in the income group of 2501–5000 TL and 20.4% (n = 37) were in the income group of 1501–2500 TL. In the intervention group, 27.1% (n = 62) of fathers had completed college or higher education, compared to 20.2% (n = 40) in the control group. For mothers, 27.7% (n = 66) in the intervention group and 26.8% (n = 53) in the control group were primary school graduates. These demographic characteristics indicate a similar distribution of age, gender, income level, and parental education between both groups.

2.3 Data collection tools

Five measurement tools were utilized to assess the effectiveness of the program: the Green Crescent Life Skills Scale (GCLSS), the Self-Efficacy for Adolescents Protecting from Drug Abuse Scale (SEAPSAS), and the Scale for Refusing Tobacco, Alcohol, and Drugs. The psychometric properties of all measurement tools were evaluated, and their reliability coefficients were deemed satisfactory (Cronbach's $\alpha > .70$) [45]. **Table 2** presents detailed information about the scales used in the study.

2.3.1 The Green Crescent Life Skills Scale (GCLS Scale)

The psychometric properties of the GCLS (in press) for middle school students were evaluated by the authors. There were four sub-dimensions of the GCLS factor loads ranging between .72 and .33, explaining 34.6% of the total variance. These subscales were: (1) self-awareness and body image (awareness of the changing body, healthy life choices); (2) coping with negative emotions (coping with negative emotions, coping with challenging life events, positive thinking, self-control); (3) thinking skills (problem-solving, critical thinking, decision-making); (4) peer relations (relationship initiation and maintenance skills, resisting peer pressure, distinguishing between safe and unsafe areas). The GCLS's four-factor model had the following goodness-of-fit indices: CFI = .98, RMSEA = .04. Besides, measurement invariance across gender indicated the GCLS was assessing the same latent structure in girls and boys.

2.3.2 Self-Efficacy Skills in Avoiding Substance Use Scale (SES-ASUS)

The SES-ASUS was developed to measure the self-efficacy of high school students for refusing drug abuse and consists of four subscales with a five-point Likert-type rating and 24 items [46]. The psychometric properties of the SES-ASUS for middle school students were evaluated by the authors. The SES-ASUS middle school version's four-factor model had the following goodness-of-fit indices: CFI = .99, RMSEA = .04. Thus, the middle school version's four-factor model had satisfactory goodness of fit. These four factors were (1) substance use avoidance, (2) resisting peer pressure on

Scales	Cronbach alpha (pre; post; follow-up)	Item number	Max score	Min score
Green Crescent Life Skills Scale (GCLSS)	.96; .97; .98	53	265	53
Self-Awareness and Body Image (SA)	.84; .86; .96	10	50	10
Coping With Negative Emotions (CNE)	.89; .92; .92	11	55	11
Thinking Skills (TS)	.91; .95; .96	14	70	14
Peer Relations (TSPR)	.91; .94; .96	18	90	18
Refusing Tobacco	.82; .83; .88	4	20	4
Refusing Alcohol	.86; .65; .89	4	20	4
Refusing Drugs	.85; .85; .90	4	20	4
Self-Efficacy Skills in Avoiding Substance Use Scale (SES-ASUS)	.94; .95; .96	23	115	23
Substance Use Avoidance (SUA)	.94; .92; .91	12	60	12
Resisting Peer Pressure on Substance Use (RPP-SU)	.73; .92; .90	4	20	4
Help-Seeking Regarding Substance-Related Issues (HS-RSRI)	.84; .85; .90	4	20	4
Supporting Friends Against Substances (SF-AS)	.70; .81; .82	3	15	3

Table 2.
Characteristics of the scales.

substance use, (3) help-seeking regarding substance-related issues, and (4) supporting friends against substances. The high total score on the scale indicated high self-efficacy skills in avoiding substance use.

2.3.3 The Refusing Tobacco, Alcohol and Substance Scales

The Refusing Tobacco, Alcohol, and Substance Scales assess the responses individuals may exhibit when confronted with such offers. According to the results of the exploratory factor analysis, the total variance explained for the Refusing Tobacco Scale was 48.29%, 48.13% for the Alcohol Scale and 50.95% for the Refusing Substance Scale. Confirmatory Factor Analysis results showed that the construct validity of all three scales was high. Specifically, the Refusing Tobacco Scale achieved goodness-of-fit indices of RMSEA = .08 and CFI = .99. Similarly, the Refusing Alcohol Scale achieved RMSEA = .042 and CFI = 1.00, while the Refusing Substance Scale achieved RMSEA = .078 and CFI = .99. The high total score of the scales indicated the high refusing skills.

2.4 GCLS program and process

The Turkish Green Crescent Society initiated the GCLS Program in Türkiye in collaboration with the Ministry of National Education (MoNE). Today, the MoNE and the Turkish Green Crescent Society manage the program jointly.

The GCLS is a universal, school-based prevention program aimed at protecting against substance use and promoting empowerment under primary prevention initiatives. The target group for the program consists of 7th-grade students who had never tried tobacco, alcohol, or drugs, or who had tried but were not regular users. The program focuses on developing basic life skills in three key areas: self-awareness and body image, coping with negative emotions, and peer relations. The program was implemented through educational games and experiential activities designed to address problem areas that the target age group might encounter in real life. The GCLS program was carried out over seven sessions, with three additional booster lessons to be delivered in the following year.

The Standards of Excellence (International Youth Foundation) of the GCLS program provides four key areas to increase the effectiveness and sustainability of life skills programs: program selection, formator training, creation of the learning environment, and monitoring evaluation. In line with these standards, a pilot study was carried out to test the program on the target audience before dissemination. In this context, the effectiveness of the GCLS program was examined in a pilot intervention study (2 × 3 mixed patterns) conducted in two schools in Istanbul, which represented a small sample of Türkiye. The program had a large impact on self-awareness, coping with negative emotions, and thinking skills, especially in the field of life skills. After the pilot study, facilitators (school psychological counselors) who delivered the program and conducted the intervention attended 5 days of training (the GCLS program format or training workshop) before the beginning of the program. The training session included detailed descriptions of the rationale for the program, aims, procedure/protocol for conducting the program, and method of data. Nine of the facilitators who completed this training conducted the intervention and data collection processes as part of the effectiveness study. The authors scheduled regular meetings to monitor and provide oversight of the school counselors' performance during the implementation of the program. Before delivery of the program, necessary permissions were obtained from the MoNE. After establishing contact with the school principals, their consent was granted for involvement in the study. Parental consent was obtained from each parent of the students in the intervention and control groups. Additionally, students were informed that they could withdraw from the study at any time.

To ensure the fidelity of program implementation, a 21-item checklist was developed based on two domains—adherence and moderating factors—suggested by Carroll et al. [47]. An average score greater than 90% (19/21) indicated that the program was feasible and reliable, a result consistent with the fidelity findings of previous life skills programs [48].

For the process evaluation of the program, the authors collected the data from the students who participated in the program and the facilitators who implemented the program through the session evaluation forms they filled out after each session. The sessions evaluation forms filled out by the students consisted of 10 questions that were scored on a 5-point Likert scale. Three of the questions were related to the benefits and content of the session, two were related to the facilitator, and five items were designed to assess the session's outcomes. During the implementation of the program, facilitators collected feedback from the students at the end of each session through session evaluation forms and reviewed this feedback. As a result of this review, the authors shared impressions during the supervision sessions at the outset, midpoint, and conclusion of the effectiveness study. Then, the authors utilized these impressions to support and enrich the program.

The session evaluation forms filled out by the facilitators consisted of 16 questions with "yes" and "no" options. Eight of the questions were related to the program's practicality, while the other eight focused on the efficiency of students' participation in the session. During the program, facilitators filled out this form at the end of each session and provided feedback to the authors during supervision meetings. The authors utilized the comprehensive feedback gathered following the effectiveness study to support and enrich the program.

2.5 Data analysis

In the study, the authors analyzed to determine the effectiveness of the GCLS program in line with two main objectives. The first objective of the study was to determine the effectiveness of the GCLS programs, and thus, the authors applied factorial ANOVA based on 2 × 3 mixed patterns to compare the changes of the intervention and control groups before and after the intervention. In this analysis, basic effect tests were performed for the group and measurement, and the main focus was on the group-measurement interaction effect test, which showed the effect of the intervention process. The authors then interpreted the interaction effect test results by considering the changes in the pretest, posttest, and follow-up test mean scores of the groups [49]. The interpretations in this study were based on the results of this test, which was the focus of the analyses. In cases where the interaction effects were significant, the authors examined the repeated measures ANOVA results on the intervention group to determine in which groups the observed change occurred and made pairwise comparisons using the Bonferroni correction. To examine the effect of statistically significant differences between the groups in practice, the authors calculated partial eta-square (η^2) effect size statistics ($\eta^2 = 0.01$ small, $\eta^2 = 0.06$ medium, and $\eta^2 = 0.14$ large effect).

3. Findings

Based on the findings of the study, the GCLS program had positive effects on Turkish adolescents' self-awareness and body image, coping with negative emotions, thinking skills, and peer relationship competencies, contributing to their overall life skills development. It was also clear that the program positively affected the self-efficacy skills in avoiding substance use. Although there was an increase in students' refusal skill scores regarding tobacco, alcohol, and substance use, these increased scores were not statistically significant.

3.1 Life skills

The mean scores and standard deviation values of the pretest, posttest, and follow-up test scores of the students from the GCLSS and its subscales are presented in **Table 3** and **Figure 1**.

Table 4 presents the mixed ANOVA and pairwise comparison results of the changes observed in the life skills of the intervention and control groups.

The study found that the life skills scores of the intervention group and control group differed significantly. In other words, the interaction effect of being in intervention and control groups and repeated measures factors on life skills was significant, $F(2, 772) = 8.518$, $p < .05$. This finding showed that the factors of being in intervention and control groups and repeated measures (pretest, posttest, follow-up test) interactively caused a significant change in life skills. To assess the effect size of the program, partial eta squared was examined, and it was determined that the program had a small effect on life skills ($\eta^2 = .022$).

Outcome	Group	Pretest			Posttest			Follow-up		
		Mean	SD	n	Mean	SD	n	Mean	SD	n
GCLS	Int.	209.7	37.3	209	231.6	30.7	209	229.3	39.9	209
	Cont.	199.4	33.4	179	205.7	42.92	179	211.0	45.5	179
SA	Int.	40.5	7.9	209	44.2	7.56	209	43.9	8.0	209
	Cont.	39.5	6.9	178	40.3	8.00	178	41.4	9.5	178
CNE	Int.	42.3	9.3	209	46.8	7.8	209	46.5	8.8	209
	Cont.	39.1	9.1	179	40.6	9.6	179	41.7	11.0	179
TSPR	Int.	54.7	11.63	208	60.6	9.3	208	60.7	10.7	208
	Cont.	52.2	9.80	177	53.7	12.6	177	55.8	12.4	177
PR	Int.	72.3	13.7	208	79.6	11.2	208	78.7	14.4	208
	Cont.	69.2	13.1	176	71.7	15.6	176	73.4	15.2	176

Table 3.
Mean and standard deviation values of the GCLSS and its subscales. SD = standard deviation, n = sample size.

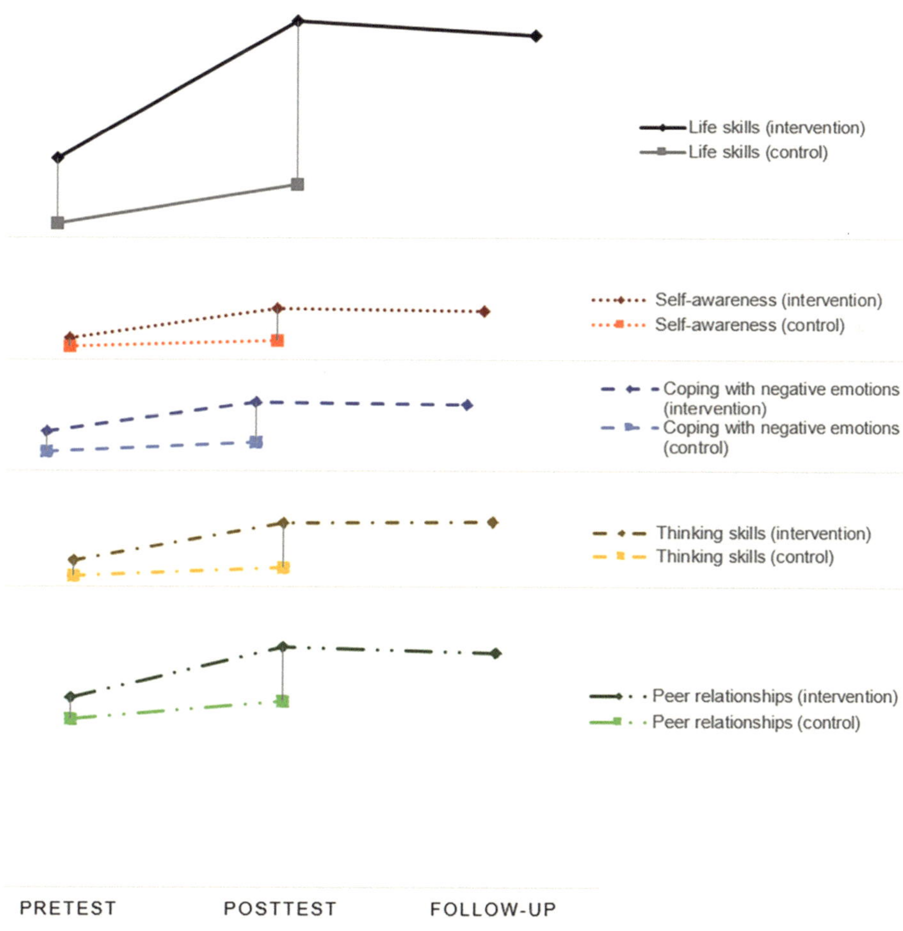

Figure 1.
Mean score changes of the GCLSS and its subscales.

Variable	Source of variance	df	F	p	η^2	MD (95% CI)	
GCLS	Between groups					*Intervention (post-pre)*	*Intervention (post-fol.)*
	Group	1	31.143	.000*	.075	21.89* (−27.8; 15.9)	2.297 (−9.01; 4.42)
	Error	386					
	Within groups						
	Measurement (pre, post, follow-up)	2	41.211	.000*	.096		
	Group*Measure	2	8.518	.000*	.022		
	Error	772					
SA	Between groups					3.699* (−5.27; 2.12)	.273 (−1.87; 1.32)
	Group	1	15.283	.000*	.038		
	Error	385					
	Within groups						
	Measurement	2	20.587	.000*	.051		
	Group*Measure	2	5.183	.006*	.013		
	Error	770					
CNE	Between groups					4.459* (−6.02; 2.88)	0.263 (−1.74; 1.21)
	Group	1	36.734	.000*	.087		
	Error	386					
	Within groups						
	Measurement	2	32.655	.000*	.078		
	Group*Measure	2	5.205	.006*	.013		
	Error	772					
TS	Between groups					5.875* (3.93; 7.81)	−.115 (−2.06; −1.83)
	Group	1	36.734	.000*	.087		
	Error	386					
	Within groups						
	Measurement	2	37.200	.000*	.089		
	Group*Measure	2	7.321	.001*	.019		
	Error	766					
PR	Between groups					7.279* (5.06; 9.49)	.923 (−3.27; 1.42)
	Group	1	21.951	.000*	.054		
	Error	382					
	Within groups						
	Measurement	2	33.822	.000*	.081		
	Group*Measure	2	5.374	.005*	.014		
	Error	764					

$^*p < 0.05$.

Table 4.
ANOVA and multiple comparison test results for GCLS and its subscales. df = degrees of freedom, F = F-test, η^2 = partial eta squared, MD = mean difference, CI = confidence interval for difference.

In addition, the authors examined the results of pairwise comparisons between the measurements in the intervention group to determine whether the program caused a significant interaction effect, and to evaluate the effect of the program. While there was a significant difference between the pretest and posttest of the intervention group (MD = 21.89, $p < .05$), the difference between the posttest and the follow-up test was not significant (MD = 2.29, $p > .05$). These findings showed that the GCLS program had a meaningful and sustainable effect on improving students' life skills. In particular, this development observed in favor of the intervention group showed that the program was effective in increasing students' life skills.

The authors also observed significant differences in the scores before and after the intervention between the intervention and control groups in terms of self-awareness, coping with negative emotions, thinking skills, and peer relationship skills. In the analysis of self-awareness skills, the interaction effect of intervention and control groups and repeated measures was significant, $F(2, 770) = 5.183$, $p < .05$. After the program, there was a significant increase in the self-awareness skills of the intervention group. Similarly, there was a significant improvement in the skills of the intervention group in terms of coping skills with negative emotions, $F(2, 772) = 5.205$, $p < .05$. Similarly, the analysis on thinking skills determined that the GCLS program made a significant contribution to students' thinking skills, $F(2, 766) = 7.231$, $p < .05$. Finally, in examinations of peer relationships, the GCLS program had a significant effect on increasing peer relationships, $F(2, 764) = 5.374$, $p < .05$. Although the effect sizes for each subscale were small, the GCLS program provided an improvement in the relevant skills (η^2; 0.013–0.019).

The results of the pairwise comparisons for the life skills subscales showed that the difference between the pretest and posttest scores of the intervention group was significant for self-awareness ($MD_{SA} = 3.69$), coping with negative emotions ($MD_{CNE} = 4.45$), thinking skills ($MD_{TS} = 5.87$), and peer relationships ($MD_{PR} = 7.27$, $p < .05$). The results also determined no significant differences between the posttest and follow-up test scores ($MD_{SA} = .273$; $MD_{CNE} = .263$; $MD_{TS} = .115$; $MD_{PR} = .923$, $p > .05$). These results showed that the GCLS program has a significant and lasting effect on improving students' self-awareness, coping with negative emotions, thinking skills, and peer relationships.

3.2 Self-efficacy skills in avoiding substance use

Table 5 presents the pretest, posttest, and follow-up test mean scores and standard deviation values obtained by the students from the SEAPSAS and its subscales (**Figure 2**).

Mixed ANOVA and pairwise comparison results regarding self-efficacy skills in avoiding substance use are given in **Table 6**.

The study found that the self-efficacy of the intervention group and the control group for avoiding substance abuse differed significantly. In other words, the interaction effect of the factors on the self-efficacy for avoiding substance abuse was significant, $F(2, 766) = 4.908$, $p < .05$. This finding showed that repeated measures factors with intervention and control groups interactively caused a significant change in self-efficacy. According to the examinations of the partial eta-square effect size values, the program had a small effect on the self-efficacy for avoiding substance abuse ($\eta^2 = .013$).

Outcomes	Group	Pretest			Posttest			Follow-up		
		Mean	SD	n	Mean	SD	n	Mean	SD	n
SES-ASUS	Intervention	100.3	19.1	211	105.7	14.1	211	103.7	19.0	211
	Control	100.8	15.8	174	100.1	20.5	174	99.7	22.4	174
SUA	Intervention	54.0	9.9	210	55.6	7.4	210	54.6	9.9	210
	Control	54.7	8.4	170	53.8	10.8	170	53.9	10.2	170
RPP-SU	Intervention	18.3	3.2	210	18.8	2.3	210	18.1	3.4	210
	Control	18.3	3.0	172	17.6	4.0	172	17.7	3.8	172
HS-RSRI	Intervention	16.4	4.3	210	18.0	3.31	210	17.7	3.9	210
	Control	15.7	4.1	172	16.5	4.50	172	16.5	4.3	172
SF-AS	Intervention	11.9	3.2	211	13.1	2.6	211	13.2	2.8	211
	Control	12.0	3.0	174	12.3	3.2	174	12.8	2.9	174

Table 5.
Mean and standard deviation values of SES-ASUS and subscales (pretest, posttest, and follow-up).
SD = standard deviation, n = sample size.

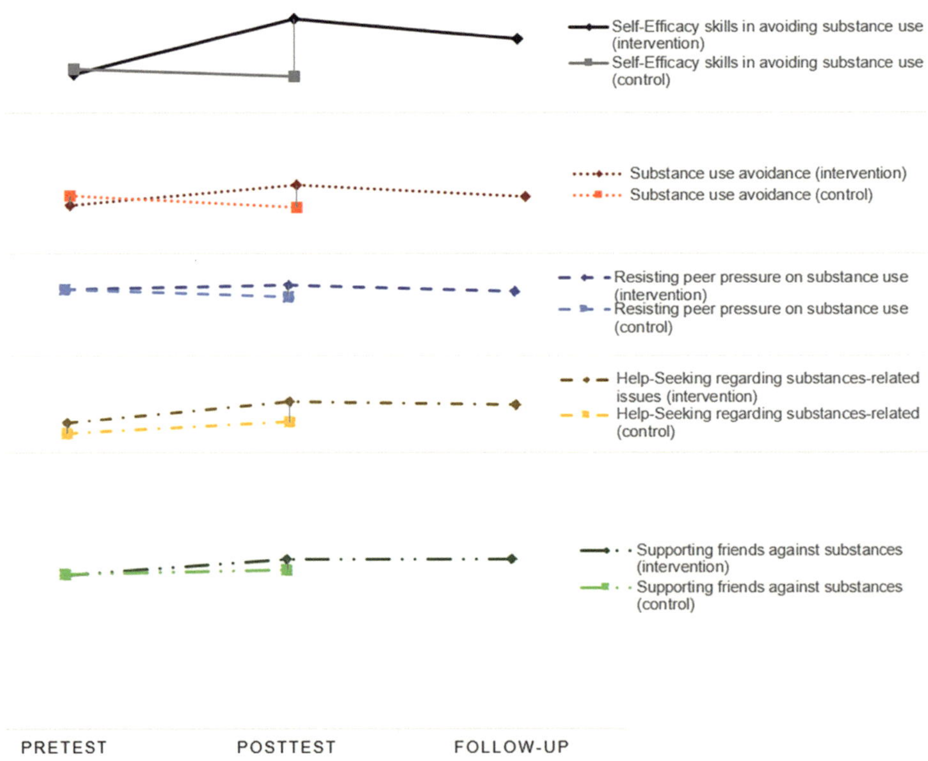

Figure 2.
Mean scores changes of SEAPSAS Scale and its subscales.

In addition, the authors examined the results of pairwise comparisons between the measurements in the intervention group to determine whether the program caused a significant interaction effect and to evaluate the effect of the program. While there was a significant difference between the pretest and posttest of the intervention group ($MD = 5.412$, $p < .05$), this finding indicated that the program was effective in

Variable	Source of variance	df	F	p	η^2	Intervention MD (95% CI)	
SES-ASUS	Between groups					*Post-pre*	*Post-follow*
	Group	1	4.131	.043		5.412* (2.64; 8.17)	2.000 (5.38; −1.38)
	Error	383					
	Within groups						
	Measurement (pre, post, follow-up)	2	2.731	.066			
	Group*Measure	2	4.908	.008	.013*		
	Error	766					
SUA	Between groups					1.648* (.273; 3.02)	1 (−2.84; .84)
	Group	1	.615	.433			
	Error	378					
	Within groups						
	Measurement	2	.379	.685			
	Group*Measure	2	3.247	.039	.009*		
	Error	756					
RPP-SU	Between groups					.457* (−.08; −1.00)	.686* (.03; 1.33)
	Group	1	4.178	.042			
	Error	380					
	Within groups						
	Measurement	2	2.593	.075			
	Group*Measure	2	4.454	.012	.012*		
	Error	760					
HS-RSRI	Between groups					—	—
	Group	1	12.832	.000			
	Error	380					
	Within groups						
	Measurement	2	16.281	.000			
	Group*Measure	2	1.493	.225			
	Error	760					
SF-AS	Between groups					1.237* (.70; 1.76)	−.047 (−.55; .46)
	Group	1	2.736	.099			
	Error	383					
	Within groups						
	Measurement	2	20.726	.000			
	Group*Measure	2	3.737	.024	.010*		
	Error	766					

*$p < 0.05$.

Table 6.
ANOVA and multiple comparison test results for SES-ASUS and subscales. df = degrees of freedom, F = F-test, η^2 = partial eta squared, MD = mean difference, CI: confidence interval for difference.

increasing students' self-efficacy in avoiding substance abuse. In addition, there was no significant difference between the posttest and follow-up test scores ($MD = 2.00$, $p > .05$). Accordingly, the GCLS program has a significant and lasting effect on increasing the self-efficacy of students for avoiding substance abuse.

The authors observed significant differences among the intervention and control groups in the scores before and after the intervention in terms of self-efficacy for avoiding substance use, supporting friends against substance use, and resisting peer pressure on substance use skills. In the analysis on self-efficacy for avoiding substance abuse, the interaction effect of being in intervention and control groups and repeated measures was significant, $F(2, 756) = 3.247$, $p < .05$. Similarly, the interaction effect was significant in terms of the supporting friends against substances, $F(2, 776) = 3.737$, $p < .05$. Finally, the interaction effect of the GCLS program on the self-efficacy for resisting peer pressure on substance use and repeated measures was significant, $F(2, 760) = 4.454$, $p < .05$. Although the effect sizes were small (η^2; 0.009–0.012), the program was effective on students' self-efficacy for avoiding substance abuse, supporting friends against substance use, and resisting peer pressure on substance use. The results showed that the self-efficacy of students in intervention and control groups did not differ significantly after the intervention, $F(2, 760) = 1.493$, $p > .05$. The program did not have a significant effect on increasing students' self-efficacy levels in seeking help regarding substance-related issues.

The results of the pairwise comparisons of the subscales in which the interaction effect was significant revealed that the pretest and posttest difference scores of the intervention groups' self-efficacy for avoiding substance abuse, supporting friends against substances, and resisting peer pressure on substance use were significant ($MD_{ADU} = 1.648$, $p < .05$; $MD_{PSU\text{-}FRSU} = 1.237$, $p < .05$; $MD_{RDU\text{-}UP} = .45$, $p < .05$). According to the results of the follow-up test, the differences between the posttest and follow-up test scores regarding the self-efficacy for substance use and supporting friends against substance after the program were not significant ($MD_{ADU} = 1$, $p > .05$; $MD_{PSU\text{-}FRSU} = .047$, $p > .05$). Accordingly, this finding showed that the program had a significant and lasting effect on these two subscales. This finding showed that the program did not have a lasting effect on the self-efficacy for resisting peer pressure on substance use ($MD_{RDU\text{-}UP} = .686$, $p < .05$).

3.3 Skills of refusing tobacco, alcohol and drugs

The mixed ANOVA results revealed that the changes observed in the skills of refusing tobacco, alcohol, and substances pretest, posttest, and follow-up scores did not show significant differences between the intervention and control groups. In other words, the interaction effect between the intervention and control groups and repeated measures factors was not statistically significant (F Refusing Tobacco (2.748) = 5.912, $p > .05$; F Refusing Alcohol (2.744) = 1.934, $p > .05$; F Refusing Substances (2.742) = 2.456, $p > .05$). These findings suggest that the GCLS program did not have a significant effect on improving students' skills in refusing tobacco, alcohol, and substances.

4. Discussion

This study contributes to the body of research on school-based life skills programs for preventing adolescents' tobacco, alcohol, and other substance use by introducing the evidence-based Green Crescent Life Skills Program (GCLS). This study tested the effects of the GCLS program on adolescents' life skills, self-efficacy in avoiding substance use, and substance refusal skills in a study group collected from different regions of Türkiye. As a result of the study, it was determined that the program had a significant effect on adolescents' life skills and self-efficacy in protecting against substance use.

The findings indicate that students in the intervention group exhibited significant enhancements in self-awareness, body image, coping with negative emotions, thinking skills, and peer relationship skills and that these enhancements had a positive impact. These findings support earlier research and imply that the program can be a useful instrument for helping students build life skills [39, 49–52].

Systematic literature reviews indicate that life skills programs, within the framework of addiction prevention, can influence shaping attitudes and foster the development of interpersonal skills [53–55]. Life skills have a crucial role in shaping students' self-perception, fostering a healthier body image, and equipping them with the ability to recognize and effectively regulate their behaviors, emotions, and cognitive processes [54, 55]. This awareness enhances students' abilities to identify and understand emotions, relate their feelings to thoughts and thinking styles, manage stress, relax, and develop help-seeking behaviors [53]. Individuals who know very little about themselves appear to be more affected by negative events compared to those who are confident in themselves [54]. In such cases, self-awareness and self-regulation help prevent risky behaviors [51, 55, 56], that could lead to addiction. Moreover, the development of the intrapersonal element of peer resistance skills (i.e., staying committed to a certain decision) assists students in adhering to choices they are confident about. Additionally, through thinking skills that promote informed decision-making and healthy choices in their lives, students access accurate information sources [53]. As stated by Peters and others [57], intrapersonal skills provide an important foundation for individuals to gain self-confidence.

Interpersonal skills within life skills education enhance students' abilities to establish and maintain healthy and supportive social relationships. Life skills improve students' supportive social relationships by teaching communication skills, empathy, negotiation and refusal strategies, cooperation, teamwork abilities, and techniques to motivate others to act in specific ways [53, 56]. Thus, they provide a foundation for the healthy development of peer relationships [57]. Comprehensive meta-analytic studies have revealed that school-based social and emotional learning interventions improve students' social behaviors, strengthen their relationships with peers, and enhance their social skills [51, 52].

Findings regarding the impact of the GCLS program on students' refusal skills for tobacco, alcohol, and substance use contradict this study's expected results and similar studies [58, 59] in the field as well. The GCLS program did not exhibit significant improvement in refusal skills. These findings contradict certain results in recent research on the effectiveness of school-based interventions [49, 50]. Studies generally suggest that universal, school-based prevention programs are effective in reducing substance use, though the degree of effectiveness varies based on metrics and implementation contexts. For example, programs like "LifeSkills Training (LST)" have been reported to achieve sustainable outcomes over 6.5 years, particularly in enhancing refusal skills and social competence. However, the effectiveness of such programs often depends on factors such as program duration, facilitator training, and the social influences on students [50, 60, 61].

While this study observed students' refusal skill scores for tobacco, alcohol, and substance use showed an increase, this improvement was not statistically significant.

This could be due in part to the fact that the participants' scores on the scales were extremely near the highest possible score. This result can be explained by the concept of the "ceiling effect." The ceiling effect is the situation where a measured variable reaches a high level and the measuring instrument cannot detect differences above that level. This effect makes it difficult to fully separate the performance of individuals and to detect real differences between groups. The ceiling effect occurs especially when the measuring instruments are not sensitive enough or when the performance of the sample is generally concentrated at the upper limits. In research, the ceiling effect can prevent the determination of statistical significance and the evaluation of real efficiency differences [62]. In this study, the maximum score obtained from the measurement tools used (Refusing Tobacco = 20; Refusing Alcohol = 20; Refusing Substances = 20) and the pretest scores that the students received from these scales (Refusing Tobacco = 16.39; Refusing Alcohol = 16.80; Refusing Substances = 16.98) seem to be quite close to each other. For this reason, it is thought that the most important factor in the lack of a significant effect in substance rejection is the ceiling effect [63]. There are also other prevention programs that attribute the minimal observed differences to the presence of a ceiling effect [62, 64].

In this study, students' average age was 12, and there are two primary factors that contributed to their relatively high pretest scores: (1) The possibility that the students had not yet been exposed to substances, which is consistent with the age of initial exposure reported in the literature on addictive substances [23, 65], (2) Due to the omnipotent thinking characteristic of adolescence, students may perceive themselves as capable of handling any challenge, leading to such self-reports [66]. The use of self-report scales instead of directly measuring the skills may have influenced this outcome. Fan and others [67] argue that this can be explained both by omnipotent thinking and adolescents' tendency to present themselves in a more favorable light in a classroom setting. Another possible explanation for the findings is that the group targeted for the interventions was selected randomly from across Türkiye rather than from at-risk populations. Research indicates that targeted interventions yield stronger outcomes in socioeconomically disadvantaged groups or high-risk individuals. Since the GCLS program is designed as a universal intervention, its effects may have been limited [61, 68]. One of the reasons the increase in refusal skills for alcohol, tobacco, and substances was not significant may also be related to the duration and intensity of the program. It has been reported that short programs designed to develop such skills are often insufficient to produce meaningful behavioral changes in students. For instance, longer and more comprehensive programs have been shown to be more effective [13, 68, 69].

The effectiveness of the GCLS program in enhancing students' self-efficacy in avoiding substance use, especially in areas "substance use avoidance," "resisting peer pressure on substance use," and "supporting friends against substances," is noteworthy because self-efficacy is a significant factor in substance abuse, particularly for middle school students who are searching for their identity. The program's positive impact on these specific self-efficacy skills suggests its potential in fostering long-term resistance to substance abuse [70–72], similar to other empowerment programs [73].

The increase in self-efficacy skills in substance use prevention after the GCLS program is crucial in preventing substance addiction. Studies have shown that interventions focusing on life skills can increase self-efficacy, empower individuals to make healthier choices and resist negative influences [74]. The GCLS program is a classroom-based program where students can interact with each other and build positive relationships through classmate-based activities. Building healthy relationships can be an indicator of an increase in self-efficacy in avoiding substances [75]. Self-efficacy in avoiding substances focuses on inner strength that students can use to prevent substance use [76], and since the GCLS program is based on strengths and prior success in drug refusal, we can say that increased awareness of inner strength increases self-sufficiency skills.

The GCLS program was found to significantly increase students' capacity to avoid substance use. The increased knowledge and awareness brought about by the program could be considered one of the causes of this [61, 77]. Life skills can effectively build young adults' empowerment and self-competence [74]. In the course of the program, students were asked to identify their life skills and attempt to link them to the skills that would help them avoid substances and drugs. Additionally, they might become more confident and better understand their own values and objectives [53, 78]. As a result, they were better equipped to make decisions that supported their own health, such as abstaining from substances.

Additionally, it was noted that the program improved their capacity to resist peer pressure on substance use. This result also aligns with the program's goal of helping students become more adept at gaining the ability to regulate peer relations. It is possible that the program may have equipped students with assertiveness training and communication skills, especially in peer relations, enabling them to express their opinions and refuse unwanted offers more confidently since the program has components where students could be able to express their opinions and skills [77]. Their increased sense of self-efficacy in resisting peer pressure to use substances is probably influenced by their newly discovered capacity for self-assertion [39, 43, 79]. As their self-esteem grows, they might become less dependent on outside approval and better equipped to resist peer pressure to abuse substances [78].

The GCLS program also yielded significant results in students supporting their friends against substances, which can also be the result of the focus of the program on regulating peer relations. The content of the program included activities where students shared their own coping strategies, listened to each other, supported each other, and worked with their friends, allowing students to develop skills that would help them avoid substances and support their friends in staying away from drugs [80]. Also, in substance prevention programs, it is very important to have support from friends and family [81, 82]. Therefore, the fact that the GCLS program significantly increases friend support against substance use can be considered a valuable finding for the literature.

However, the GCLS program did not significantly affect the help-seeking skills regarding substance-related issues. Similar to the changes in students' refusal skill scores for tobacco, alcohol, and substance use, this could be attributed to pre-existing high levels of help seeking in this area among the students. The minimum score that students can get in help-seeking drug use skills is 4, and the maximum score is 20. The students' mean score was 16.26 before the GCLS program, but it rose to 17.56 after. The main factor in the lack of significant change here can be defined as the floor-ceiling effect [63]. It is important to acknowledge that the effectiveness of interventions may vary depending on the specific skills being targeted and the baseline levels of help-seeking regarding substance use within the target population [58, 83, 84]. In addition, in this phase of development, the source of help for adolescents could be their friends. They seek help from their peers even before seeking help from authorities like teachers or social workers [85]. In other words, since friends are already a source of help-seeking in this developmental phase, it may explain why participants' help-seeking regarding substance use scores were high before the program.

5. Conclusion and suggestions

In this study, we found that implementation of an evidence-based life skills program to prevent alcohol, tobacco, and substance use in Türkiye had positive effects on self-awareness, coping with negative emotions, thinking skills and peer relations, life skills, and self-efficacy for protecting substance abuse among Turkish adolescents. Promoting self-sufficiency skills through targeted interventions can play a significant role in preventing substance addiction. By empowering individuals to resist peer pressure, make informed decisions, and seek help when needed, these interventions can contribute to building healthier and more resilient communities. However, it is essential to tailor interventions to the specific needs of the target population and consider their existing levels of self-sufficiency across different domains. In this study, the limited effects of the GCLS program on the ability to refuse alcohol, tobacco, and substance use were observed, suggesting modifications in future interventions. Strategies such as longer-term implementation, targeted interventions, and the strengthening of social support components could increase the effectiveness of the program. The GCLS program targets only 7th-grade students, which may limit its impact due to the absence of critical factors such as family involvement [86]. Since studies like Eisen and others [87] and Konkel [88] have highlighted the value of family-based interventions in preventing substance use, it is well known that this component increases student engagement with program content. Additionally, considering pretest scores when assessing the program's impact, utilizing behavioral measurement tools, and replicating the study with more specialized samples could make significant contributions to substance use. The findings of this study have assessed the effects of the program developed for 7th-grade students through pretests, posttests, and follow-up tests. However, to fully understand the long-term effects of behavioral changes in students, further research is necessary. For instance, by including a randomized control trial, it would be possible to conduct a more thorough investigation into the program's effectiveness. Also, longitudinal studies are recommended to examine the continuity and impact of behavioral changes in greater depth. Such studies would allow for a clearer understanding of how students undergo behavioral transformations over time due to the program, thereby providing a broader perspective on the effectiveness of the programs. Furthermore, because attitudinal aspects require more experience and changes take longer to manifest, longitudinal research will make it easier to observe long-term predicted changes in variables. Another important thing is that the use of self-report scales in these kinds of studies may be a limitation because genuine responses might not be provided due to appearance anxiety or the fear of a disciplinary action from the school administration for substance use, if it exists. It might be advised to include observational data when assessing the studies' efficacy.

Acknowledgements

The development and effectiveness evaluation process of the program addressed in this study was funded by the Turkish Green Crescent Society, and the human and physical resources required for implementation were provided by the Ministry of National Education. However, no financial or human resources were provided by the relevant organizations during the publication phase.

Author details

A. Esra Ismen Gazioglu[1*], Seher Merve Erus[2], Cigdem Demir Celebi[3], Neslihan Yaman[4], Derya Eryigit[5], Bilge Nuran Aydogdu[6], Halime Yildirim Hos[7] and Seyma Arslan[8]

1 Istanbul University-Cerrahpaşa, Istanbul, Turkey

2 Yıldız Technical University, Istanbul, Turkey

3 Istanbul Sabahattin Zaim University, Istanbul, Turkey

4 Yalova University, Yalova, Turkey

5 Marmara University, Istanbul, Turkey

6 Balıkesir University, Balıkesir, Turkey

7 Istanbul Medeniyet University, Istanbul, Turkey

8 Ministry of National Education, Istanbul, Turkey

*Address all correspondence to: ismen@iuc.edu.tr

References

[1] Llistosella M, Castellví P, García-Ortiz M, López-Hita G, Torné C, Ortiz R, et al. Effectiveness of a resilience school-based intervention in adolescents at risk: A cluster-randomized controlled trial. Frontiers in Psychology. 2024;**15**:1-11. DOI: 10.3389/fpsyg.2024.1478424

[2] Simon DJ. School-Centered Interventions: Evidence-Based Strategies for Social, Emotional, and Academic Success. Washington, DC: American Psychological Association; 2016. DOI: 10.1037/14779-000

[3] Santiago CD, Raviv T, Jaycox LH. Creating Healing School Communities: School-Based Interventions for Students Exposed to Trauma. Washington, DC: American Psychological Association; 2018

[4] Werner-Seidler A, Perry Y, Calear AL, Newby JM, Christensen H. School-based depression and anxiety prevention programs for young people: A systematic review and meta-analysis. Clinical Psychology Review. 2017;**51**:30-47. DOI: 10.1016/j.cpr.2016.10.005

[5] World Health Organization. Skills for Health: Skills-Based Health Education, Including Life Skills: An Important Component of a Child-Friendly/Health Promoting School. Geneva: World Health Organization; 2003. Available from: https://iris.who.int/handle/10665/42818

[6] Brown GK, Owens J, Richards C, Di Folco S, Schwannauer M. Facilitators and barriers to the implementation of a school-based intervention for anxiety. Child Psychiatry and Human Development. 2023:1-12. DOI: 10.1007/s10578-023-01615-9

[7] Faggiano F, Vigna-Taglianti F, Versino E, Zambon A, Borraccino A, Lemma P. School-based prevention for illicit drug use: A systematic review. Preventive Medicine. 2008;**46**(5):385-396. DOI: 10.1016/j.ypmed.2007.11.012

[8] Gardner LA, Rowe AL, Newton NC, Egan L, Hunter E, Devine EK, et al. A systematic review and meta-analysis of school-based preventive interventions targeting e-cigarette use among adolescents. Prevention Science. 2024;**25**(7):1-5. DOI: 10.1007/s11121-024-01730-6

[9] Caulkins JP, Pacula RL, Paddock SM, Chiesa J. School-Based Drug Prevention: What Kind of Drug Use Does it Prevent? Santa Monica, CA: RAND Corporation; 2002

[10] Thomas RE, McLellan J, Perera R. School-based programmes for preventing smoking. Evidence-Based Child Health. 2013;**8**:1616-2040. DOI: 10.1002/ebch.1937

[11] Bangert-Drowns RL. The effects of school-based substance abuse education: A meta-analysis. Journal of Drug Education. 1988;**18**(3):243-264

[12] Forman SG, Linney JA, Brondino MJ. Effects of coping skills training on adolescents at risk for substance use. Psychology of Addictive Behaviors. 1990;**4**(2):67-76

[13] Griffin KW, Botvin GJ. Evidence-based interventions for preventing substance use disorders in adolescents. Child and Adolescent Psychiatric Clinics of North America. 2010;**19**(3):505-526. DOI: 10.1016/j.chc.2010.03.005

[14] Botvin GJ, Kantor LW. Preventing alcohol and tobacco use through life skills training. Alcohol Research and Health. 2000;**24**(4):250-257

[15] McGuire WJ. The nature of attitudes and attitude change. In: Lindzey G, Aronson E, editors. Handbook of Social Psychology. Oxford, England: Addison-Wesley; 1968. pp. 136-314

[16] Evans RI. Smoking in children: Developing a social psychological strategy of deterrence. Preventive Medicine. 1976;**5**(2):122-127

[17] Carson KV, Brinn MP, Labiszewski NA. Community interventions for preventing smoking in young people. Cochrane Database of Systematic Reviews. 2011;7:2-4. :CD001291. DOI: 10.1002/14651858. CD001291.pub2

[18] Thomas RE, Baker P, Thomas BC, Lorenzetti DL. Family-based programmes for preventing smoking by children and adolescents. Cochrane Database of Systematic Reviews. 2015;**2015**(2):CD004493. DOI: 10.1002/14651858.CD004493.pub2

[19] Swendsen J, Burstein M, Case B, Conway KP, Dierker L, He JP, et al. Use and abuse of alcohol and illicit drugs in U.S. adolescents: Results of the National Comorbidity Survey Adolescent Supplement. Archives of General Psychiatry. 2012;**69**(4):390-398

[20] Vega WA, Aguilar-Gaxiola S, Andrade L, Bijl R, Borges G, Caraveo-Anduaga JJ, et al. Prevalence and age of onset for drug use in seven international sites: Results from the International Consortium of Psychiatric Epidemiology. Drug and Alcohol Dependence. 2002;**68**(3):285-297. DOI: 10.1016/S0376-8716(02)00224-7

[21] Türkiye Uyuşturucu ve Uyuşturucu Bağımlılığı İzleme Merkezi-TUBİM. Avrupa Uyuşturucu ve Uyuşturucu Bağımlılığı Izleme Merkezi Ulusal Raporu [European Monitoring Center for Drugs and Drug Addiction National Report]. Ankara: Kom; 2013

[22] Avşar G, Koç F, Aslan G. Social support and self-esteem in substance addicted patients. Acıbadem University Health Sciences Journal. 2016;**1**:44-49

[23] Bilaç Ö, Kavurma C, Önder A, Doğan Y, Uzunoğlu G, Ozan E. Bir bölge ruh sağlığı hastanesi çocuk ve ergen yataklı servisinde madde kullanımı nedeniyle yatarak tedavi gören gençlerin klinik ve sosyodemografik özellikleri. Klinik Psikiyatri Dergisi. 2019;**22**:463-471

[24] Alikaşifoğlu M, Erginöz E, Ercan O, Uysal Ö, Albayrak-Kaymak D, İlter Ö. Alcohol drinking behaviors among Turkish high school students. The Turkish Journal of Pediatrics. 2004;**46**:44-53

[25] Ogel K, Tamar D, Evren C, Cakmak D. Prevalence of cigarette, alcohol, and substance use among high school youth. Türk Psikiyatri Dergisi. 2001;**12**(2):47-52

[26] Hibell B, Andersson B, Bjarnason R, Kokkevi A, Morgan M, Narusk A. The 1995 European School Survey Project on Alcohol and Other Drugs (ESPAD): Alcohol and other drug use among students in 26 European countries. Stockholm: The Swedish Council for Information on Alcohol and Other Drugs; 1997

[27] Ayvasik HB, Sümer HC. Individual differences as predictors of illicit drug use among Turkish college students. The Journal of Psychology. 2010;**144**(6):489-505. DOI: 10.1080/00223980.2010.496671

[28] Erdem G, Eke CY, Ogel K, Taner S. Peer characteristics and substance use among high school students. Journal of Dependence. 2006;7(3):111-116

[29] Ogel K, Corapcioglu A, Sir A, Tamar M, Tot S, Dogan O, et al. The prevalence of tobacco, alcohol, and substance use among elementary and secondary school students in nine cities of Turkey. Türk Psikiyatri Dergisi. 2004;**15**(2):112-118

[30] Ogel K, Taner S, Eke CY. The prevalence of tobacco, alcohol and substance use among 10th grade students: Istanbul sample. Journal of Dependence. 2006;7(1):18-23

[31] Akkuş D, Eker F, Karaca A, Kapısız Ö, Açıkgöz F. Lise Gençlerinde Akran Eğitimi Programı Madde Bağımlılığını Önlemede Etkili Bir Model Olabilir Mi? Journal of Psychiatric Nursing. 2016;7(1):34-44. DOI: 10.5505/phd.2016.59489

[32] Albayrak S, Balci S. The prevention of drug abuse in young adults. Journal for Training and Research in Nursing. 2014;**2**:30-37

[33] Terakye G, Öz F, Üstün B. Madde bağımlılığını önleme projesi. Ankara: Yayınlanmamış araştırma raporu; 2000

[34] Canel AN, Yılmaz S, Bacanlı H, Akyılmaz FD. Training program on addiction prevention of Turkey (TBM): Content and process. Gavin Journal of Addiction Research and Therapy. 2016;**1**:29-35

[35] Türkiye Uyuşturucu ve Uyuşturucu Bağımlılığı İzleme Merkezi-TUBİM. Türkiye Uyuşturucu Raporu [Turkey Drug Report]. Ankara: EGM; 2019

[36] Aydoğdu-Sevgi M, Ögel K, Tarı-Cömert I, Yılmazçetin-Eke C. Günebakan madde bağımlılığını önleme eğitim programı. İstanbul: Yeniden Sağlık ve Eğitim Derneği; 2007. pp. 11-13

[37] Davaslıgil Ü, Çakıcı M, Ögel K. Bağımlılık ve gençlik komisyonu eğitici kılavuzu. İstanbul: İl Milli Eğitim Müdürlüğü; 1998

[38] Siyez MD, Palabıyık A. Günebakan madde bağımlılığını önleme eğitim programının lise öğrencilerinin madde kullanım sıklığı, uyuşturucu maddeler hakkındaki bilgi düzeyleri ve yanlış inanışları ile madde reddetme becerileri üzerindeki etkisi. Elektronik Sosyal Bilimler Dergisi. 2009;**8**(28):56-67

[39] Botvin GJ, Griffin KW. Life skills training: Preventing substance misuse by enhancing individual and social competence. New Directions for Youth Development. 2014;**2014**(141):57-65. DOI: 10.1002/yd.20086

[40] CASEL. Effective Social and Emotional Learning Programs. Preschool and Elementary School Edition. 2013. Available from: www.casel.org/research#Lib

[41] Giannotta F, Weichold K. Evaluation of a life skills program to prevent adolescent alcohol use in two European countries: One-year follow-up. Child & Youth Care Forum. 2016;**45**:607-624. DOI: 10.1007/s10566-016-9349-y

[42] Pan W, Bai H. A multivariate approach to a meta-analytic review of the effectiveness of the DARE program. International Journal of Environmental Research and Public Health. 2009;**6**(1):267-277. DOI: 10.3390/ijerph6010267

[43] Weichold K, Tomasik MJ, Silbereisen RK, Spaeth M. The effectiveness of the life skills program IPSY for the prevention of adolescent tobacco use: The mediating role of yielding to peer pressure. Journal of Early Adolescence. 2016;**36**(7):881-908. DOI: 10.1177/0272431615589349

[44] Botvin GJ, Griffin KW. Life skills training: Empirical findings and future

directions. The Journal of Primary Prevention. 2004;**25**:211-232

[45] Nunnally JC, Bernstein IH. Psychometric Theory. 3rd ed. New York: McGraw-Hill; 1994

[46] Eker F, Akkuş D, Kapısız Ö. Ergenler İçin Madde Bağımlılığından Korunma Öz-Yeterlik Ölçeği'nin Geliştirilmesi ve Psikometrik Değerlendirilmesi. Journal of Psychiatric Nursing/Psikiyatri Hemşireleri Derneği. 2013;**4**(1):7-12. DOI: 10.5505/phd.2013.74936

[47] Carroll C, Patterson M, Wood S, Booth A, Rick J, Balain S. A conceptual framework for implementation fidelity. Implementation Science. 2007;**2**(1):1-9. DOI: 10.1186/1748-5908-2-40

[48] Mihalic SF, Fagan AA, Argamaso S. Implementing the Life Skills Training drug prevention program: Factors related to implementation fidelity. Implementation Science. 2008;**3**(1):5. DOI: 10.1186/1748-5908-3-5

[49] Botvin GJ, Griffin KW, Botvin C, Murphy M, Acevedo B. Increasing implementation fidelity for school-based drug abuse prevention: Effectiveness of enhanced training and technical assistance. Journal of the Society for Social Work and Research. 2018;**9**(4):599-613

[50] Botvin GJ, Griffin KW. Life Skills Training: A competence enhancement approach to tobacco, alcohol, and drug abuse prevention. In: Scheier LM, editor. Handbook of Adolescent Drug Use Prevention: Research, Intervention Strategies, and Practice. Washington, DC: American Psychological Association; 2015. pp. 177-196. DOI: 10.1037/14550-011

[51] Durlak JA, Weissberg RP, Dymnicki AB, Taylor RD, Schellinger KB. The impact of enhancing students' social and emotional learning: A meta-analysis of school-based universal interventions. Child Development. 2011;**82**(1):405-432. DOI: 10.1111/j.1467-8624.2010.01564

[52] Taylor RD, Oberle E, Durlak JA, Weissberg RP. Promoting positive youth development through school-based social and emotional learning interventions: A meta-analysis of follow-up effects. Child Development. 2017;**88**(4):1156-1171. DOI: 10.1111/cdev.12864

[53] Kirchhoff E, Keller R. Age-specific life skills education in school: A systematic review. Frontiers in Education. 2021;**6**:660878. DOI: 10.3389/feduc.2021.660878

[54] Leiblein T, Bitzer E-M, Spörhase U. What skills do addiction-specific school-based life skills programs promote? Sustainability. 2022;**14**(22):15234. DOI: 10.3390/su142215234

[55] Moulier V, Guinet H, Kovacevic Z, Bel-Abbass Z, Benamara Y, Zile N, et al. Effects of a life-skills-based prevention program on self-esteem and risk behaviors in adolescents: A pilot study. BMC Psychology. 2019;**7**(82):1-10. DOI: 10.1186/s40359-019-0358-0

[56] Madsen OJ. Life Skills and Adolescent Mental Health: Can Kids be Taught to Master Life? London and New York: Routledge Taylor & Francis; 2023. DOI: 10.4324/9781003372547

[57] Peters LW, Kok G, Ten Dam GT, Buijs GJ, Paulussen TG. Effective elements of school health promotion across behavioral domains: A systematic review of reviews. BMC Public Health. 2009;**9**(1):182. DOI: 10.1186/1471-2458-9-182

[58] Butzer B, LoRusso A, Shin SH, Khalsa SBS. Evaluation of yoga for

preventing adolescent substance use risk factors in a middle school setting: A preliminary group-randomized controlled trial. Journal of Youth and Adolescence. 2017;**46**:603-632. DOI: 10.1007/s10964-016-0513-3

[59] Seal N. Preventing tobacco and drug use among Thai high school students through life skills training. Nursing and Health Sciences. 2006;**8**(3):164-168. DOI: 10.1111/j.1442-2018.2006.00275.x

[60] Fishbein DH, Sloboda Z. A National Strategy for preventing substance and opioid use disorders through evidence-based prevention programming that fosters healthy outcomes in our youth. Clinical Child and Family Psychology Review. 2023;**26**(1):1-16. DOI: 10.1007/s10567-022-00420-5

[61] Tremblay M, Baydala L, Khan M, Currie C, Morley K, Burkholder C, et al. Primary substance use prevention programs for children and youth: A systematic review. Pediatrics. 2020;**146**(3):1-22. DOI: 10.1542/peds.2019-2747

[62] Andrade C. The ceiling effect, the floor effect, and the importance of active and placebo control arms in randomized controlled trials of an investigational drug. Indian Journal of Psychological Medicine. 2021;**43**(4):360-361. DOI: 10.1177/02537176211021280

[63] Šimkovic M, Träuble B. Robustness of statistical methods when measure is affected by ceiling and/or floor effect. PLoS ONE. 2019;**14**(8):e0220889. DOI: 10.1371/journal.pone.0220889

[64] Butzer B, Ahmed K, Khalsa SBS. Yoga enhances positive psychological states in young adult musicians. Applied Psychophysiology and Biofeedback. 2016;**41**:191-202. DOI: 10.1007/s10484-015-9321-x

[65] Fırat M, Kanbay Y, Ayran G. Sigara, alkol ve madde kullanımı tarama testinin Türkçe geçerlilik ve güvenilirliği. ADDICTA: The Turkish Journal on Addictions. 2019;**6**(4):244-256. DOI: 10.5152/addicta.2020.19106

[66] Santrock JW. Yaşam Boyu Gelişim: Gelişim Psikolojisi. Ankara: Nobel; 2023

[67] Fan X, Miller BC, Park KE, Winward BW, Christensen M, Grotevant HD, et al. An exploratory study about inaccuracy and invalidity in adolescent self-report surveys. Field Methods. 2006;**18**(3):223-244

[68] Public Health Ontario. Rapid Review: Effectiveness of Interventions to Prevent Youth Substance Use. 2020. Available from: https://www.publichealthontario.ca

[69] Sussman S, Sun P, Rohrbach LA, Spruijt-Metz D. One-year outcomes of a drug abuse prevention program for older teens and emerging adults: Evaluating a motivational interviewing booster component. Health Psychology. 2012;**31**(4):476-485. DOI: 10.1037/a0025756

[70] Karatay G, Baş NG. Factors affecting substance use and self-efficacy status of students in eastern Turkey. Ciência & Saúde Coletiva. 2019;**24**:1317-1326. DOI:10.1590/1413-81232018244.30252017

[71] Karl S. The intersection of childhood trauma and addiction. Counseling Today. 2021;**63**(10):1-13. Available from: https://ct.counseling.org/2021/04/the-intersection-of-childhood-trauma-and-addiction/

[72] Sayed HA, Elwahab EL, Rasmia AE, Sattar A, Ahmed FM, Hedya FM. The effect of life skills intervention on social self-efficacy for prevention of drug abuse among young adolescent students

at Benha City. American Journal of Nursing Science. 2019;**8**(5):263-273. DOI: 10.11648/j.ajns.20190805.19

[73] Uyaroğlu AK, Özcan A. The effect of empowerment training in protecting adolescents from substance abuse on self-efficacy, self-esteem, and assertiveness levels. ADDICTA: The Turkish Journal on Addictions. 2022;**9**(3):269-276. DOI: 10.5152/ADDICTA.2022.22007

[74] Poole ME, Evans GT. Adolescents' self-perceptions of competence in life skill areas. Journal of Youth and Adolescence. 1989;**18**(2):147-173. DOI: 10.1007/BF02138798

[75] Kayaoğlu K, Özer D. Analyzing the relationship between self-efficacy in protecting against substance use and loneliness in adolescents: A cross-sectional survey. Journal of Psychosocial Nursing and Mental Health Services. 2024;**62**(9):29-36. DOI: 10.3928/02793695-20240322-02

[76] Bandura A. Self-Efficacy in Changing Societies. Cambridge: Cambridge University Press; 1997

[77] Botvin GJ, Tortu S. Preventing adolescent substance abuse through life skills training. In: Price RH, Cowen EL, Lorion RP, Ramos-McKay J, editors. Fourteen Ounces of Prevention: A Casebook for Practitioners. Washington, DC: American Psychological Association; 1988. pp. 98-110

[78] Velasco V, Cominelli S, Scattola P, Celata C. Life skill education at the time of COVID-19: Perceptions and strategies of Italian expert school educators. Health Education Research. 2021;**36**(6):615-633. DOI: 10.1093/her/cyab037

[79] Shrestha S, Velayudhan B, Shashidhara YN, Khattri JB. Effectiveness of School-based Substance abuse Prevention Programme (SSPP) on awareness, attitude, peer pressure, and life skills among adolescents in selected public schools of Pokhara, Nepal—A cluster randomized trial protocol. Mental Health & Prevention. 2024;**34**:200342. DOI: 10.1016/j.mhp.2024.200342

[80] Tuttle J, Campbell-Heider N, David TM. Positive adolescent life skills training for high-risk teens: Results of a group intervention study. Journal of Pediatric Health Care. 2006;**20**(3):184-191. DOI: 10.1016/j.pedhc.2005.10.011

[81] Branstetter SA, Low S, Furman W. The influence of parents and friends on adolescent substance use: A multidimensional approach. Journal of Substance Use. 2011;**16**(2):150-160. DOI: 10.3109/14659891.2010.519421

[82] Kail BL, Litwak E. Family, friends and neighbors: The role of primary groups in preventing the misuse of drugs. Journal of Drug Issues. 1989;**19**(2):261-281. DOI: 10.1177/002204268901900 2

[83] Rowe SL, French RS, Henderson C, Ougrin D, Slade M, Moran P. Help-seeking behaviour and adolescent self-harm: A systematic review. The Australian and New Zealand Journal of Psychiatry. 2014;**48**(12):1083-1095. DOI: 10.1177/0004867414555718

[84] Shek DT, Yu L, Leung H, Wu FK, Law MY. Development, implementation, and evaluation of a multi-addiction prevention program for primary school students in Hong Kong: The BEST Teen Program. Asian Journal of Gambling Issues and Public Health. 2016;**6**:1-17. DOI: 10.1186/s40405-016-0014-z

[85] Boldero J, Fallon B. Adolescent help-seeking: What do they get help for and from whom? Journal of Adolescence. 1995;**18**(2):193-209. DOI: 10.1006/jado.1995.1013

[86] Kumpfer KL, Alvarado R, Whiteside HO. Family-based interventions for substance use and misuse prevention. Substance Use and Misuse. 2003;**38**(11-13):1759-1787. DOI: 10.1081/JA-120024240

[87] Eisen M, Zellman GL, Murray DM. Evaluating the effectiveness of school-based drug education programs. Addictive Behaviors. 2003;**28**(5):883-897. DOI: 10.1016/S0306-4603(01)00292-1

[88] Konkel KE. Is a life skills training infusion an effective strategy to reduce substance use among at-risk teens in a mentoring program? [doctoral dissertation]. Colorado State University; 2016

Chapter 3

Emerging Therapeutic Applications for Treating Methamphetamine Use Disorder

Tuanthon Boonlue

Abstract

Methamphetamine use disorder (MUD) poses a severe global health challenge, characterized by high addiction potential, neurotoxicity, and significant societal impacts. Despite the rising prevalence of methamphetamine consumption and its intersection with the opioid crisis, effective treatment options remain limited. Current therapies focus on behavioral interventions such as cognitive-behavioral therapy and contingency management, yet retention and long-term success are challenging. Emerging pharmacological treatments, including dopaminergic agents and glutamatergic modulators, offer promise but require further investigation. Neurostimulation techniques, such as repetitive transcranial magnetic stimulation and transcranial direct current stimulation, have shown potential in reducing cravings and improving cognitive control. Novel strategies like immunotherapy and personalized interventions guided by neuroimaging and epigenetic insights represent future directions. This chapter highlights the need for integrated, multimodal approaches combining pharmacological, behavioral, and neurostimulation therapies to address the complex neurobiological and psychosocial dimensions of MUD. Advances in research, coupled with policy and healthcare collaborations, are essential to mitigate the impact of this pervasive disorder.

Keywords: methamphetamine use disorder, addiction treatment, neurostimulation, behavioral therapy, pharmacological interventions, cognitive-behavioral therapy, contingency management

1. Introduction

Methamphetamine use disorder (MUD) poses a substantial challenge to public health and is characterized by high rates of relapse, severe neurotoxicity, and increased mortality rate. In the wake of the opioid crisis, methamphetamine has re-emerged as a major challenge for mental health providers and researchers. Methamphetamine (MA) is now available in various forms, including ice, powder, and pills, each with distinct pharmacokinetic properties that contribute to its appeal among specific user populations. Recent seizure data suggest that MA production and trafficking are expanding into new global regions. Alarmingly, MA consumption increased fourfold between

2015 and 2016, and total stimulant usage doubled over the last decade [1]. Notably, there are no FDA-approved medications specifically for MUD. Existing treatments primarily focus on behavioral therapies, yet the high rates of attrition and limited effectiveness underscore the need for novel approaches [2]. This chapter examines emerging therapeutic applications for MUD, emphasizing innovative pharmacotherapies, behavioral therapies, and advancements in neurostimulation techniques.

A systematic search was conducted to identify publications focusing on emerging approaches to managing of MA use and MUD. The search was performed using the following electronic databases: PubMed, Scopus, Web of Science, and PsycINFO. The search strategy utilized a combination of MeSH terms and keywords, including but not limited to: "methamphetamine," "amphetamine-type stimulants," "treatment," "management," "behavioral therapy," "pharmacotherapy," and "psychostimulant dependence." Boolean operators ("AND," "OR") were applied to refine the search. Titles and abstracts of retrieved articles were screened for relevance. Full-text articles were then reviewed based on focusing on this topic. This structured approach ensured the inclusion of high-quality, relevant studies to provide a comprehensive review of emerging management strategies for methamphetamine use disorder.

2. Epidemiology and impact of MUD

Methamphetamine and amphetamine use continue to pose significant global health challenges. According to the United Nations Office on Drugs and Crime (UNODC), the annual prevalence of amphetamine-type stimulants (ATS), which includes MA, varies across regions. In North America, the prevalence is estimated at 2.02% of the population, while in East and Southeast Asia, it is approximately 0.6%. Notably, the prevalence in Oceania is among the highest, at 1.34% [3]. Recent trends indicate an increase in MA use in regions such as North America, East and Southeast Asia, and parts of the Middle East. Recent attention has highlighted the increasing contribution of psychostimulants, particularly MA, to overdose deaths in the United States. MA is a highly addictive and potent stimulant associated with significant physical and mental health risks, including overdose and mortality. The growing MA crisis is further complicated by its intersection with the ongoing opioid overdose epidemic. Data reveal that the involvement of opioids in psychostimulant-related overdose deaths rose dramatically from 34.5% in 2010 to 53.5% in 2019—an increase exceeding 50% [4]. MA use remains a significant issue in Australia, characterized by its widespread availability, increasing rates of use, and substantial societal impacts. Crystal MA, often imported from countries such as the United States, Mexico, and Southeast Asia, is distributed locally in various forms, including small quantities like a "point" (0.1 g) or larger amounts such as an "eight ball" (3.5 g). Street-level MA is frequently adulterated with substances such as sugar, glucose, ephedrine, or ketamine, which can constitute a significant proportion of the dose. Data from the 2018 to 2019 Drug Use Monitoring in Australia survey indicate that 64% of police detainees obtained MA through personal connections, while 28% purchased it from dealers [5]. MA use is a significant public health challenge in Southeast Asia, with the region being a major hub for production and trafficking. The Golden Triangle, encompassing the border areas of Laos, Myanmar, and Thailand, is a leading source of MA in the region. Large-scale illicit production in this area has resulted in increased purity and significantly reduced prices, making MA more accessible, particularly to younger populations. In 2021, over 1 billion MA tablets were seized across East and Southeast Asia, highlighting the magnitude of the problem. A common form of MA in the region is yaba, a combination of MA and caffeine, predominantly produced in Myanmar. Yaba is widely used in countries such as Thailand and Bangladesh, with Thai youth often turning to the drug for perceived benefits such as enhancing academic performance, increasing enjoyment during leisure activities, and alleviating feelings of loneliness and isolation [6]. The reasons for MA use vary widely depending on the characteristics of the users and their underlying motivations. A systematic review of 21 studies identified key factors driving MA use, including enhancing performance, staying awake, increasing sexual performance and impulses, mitigating withdrawal effects from other substances, coping with personal or social problems, facilitating social interactions, having fun, and alleviating physical pain or discomfort. These findings highlight that MA use often serves as a maladaptive coping mechanism for various challenges. Addressing these underlying motivations requires targeted interventions, including educational efforts to inform users about the risks, strategies to manage withdrawal effectively, and supply prevention measures [7]. A scoping review of 42 studies, including 12 English and 30 Persian articles, identified individual, social, and family factors as the primary contributors to MA use. Individual factors, such as psychological vulnerabilities and coping mechanisms, were most frequently cited, followed by social influences and family dynamics [8].

MUD is associated with severe health complications, including cardiovascular damage, neurocognitive impairment, and increased susceptibility to infectious diseases. MA use among young people aged 10–24 years is associated with significant mental health outcomes, including depression, suicidal ideation, and psychosis, as well as increased mortality risks from suicide and overdose. While evidence for a link between MA use and sexually transmitted infections, including HIV, remains inconclusive, there is minimal evidence supporting associations with dental diseases [9]. A systematic review and meta-analysis examining the health, functional, and cognitive outcomes of MA use in young people identified the strongest association with conduct disorder, with users being 13 times more likely to meet diagnostic criteria compared to non-users. MA use in youth is also linked to higher rates of justice system involvement, violence perpetration, and educational challenges. Consistent cognitive impairments, particularly in inhibitory control, have been observed in this population. However, the current body of research is limited by inconsistencies in exposure and outcome measurements, insufficient control groups, and a lack of longitudinal studies, underscoring the need for more rigorous research to elucidate the long-term effects of MA use in young people [10].

MA use is significantly associated with an increased risk of depression, as shown by a systematic review and meta-analysis. Cross-sectional studies revealed an odds ratio (OR) of 1.66, and longitudinal studies showed an OR of 1.18 for depressive outcomes among MA users. Individuals with MUD exhibited even higher odds of depression (OR = 2.80). The analysis suggests a low-to-moderate risk of unmeasured confounding, as indicated by E-values ranging from 1.28 to 6.30 [11]. Methamphetamine-induced psychosis (MIP) presents clinical features that significantly overlap with schizophrenia, complicating their differentiation. A systematic review and meta-analysis of 12 studies, involving 624 individuals with MIP and 524 individuals with schizophrenia, revealed no significant differences in positive symptoms between the groups. However, individuals with MIP exhibited significantly fewer negative symptoms compared to those with schizophrenia, suggesting potential differences in underlying neurobiological mechanisms. Despite these findings, limitations such as the cross-sectional design, variability in study populations, inclusion criteria, and drug exposure hinder causal interpretations [12]. MA use is strongly associated with adverse mental health outcomes beyond depression and psychosis. A systematic review and meta-analysis of 149 studies, including 59 in meta-analyses, found that any amphetamine use significantly increased the odds of psychosis (OR = 2.0), violence (OR = 2.2), and suicidality (OR = 4.4). For individuals with amphetamine use disorder, the risks were even higher, with increased odds of psychosis (OR = 3.0), violence (OR = 6.2), and suicidality (OR = 2.3). While most evidence comes from cross-sectional studies, these findings highlight MA use as a major risk factor for poor mental health [13]. MUD is associated with significant cognitive deficits, as evidenced by a meta-analysis of 44 studies involving 1592 individuals with MUD and 1820 healthy controls. Moderate impairments were observed across several cognitive domains, including attention, executive functions, language/verbal fluency, verbal learning and memory, visual memory, and working memory. Notably, deficits in impulsivity/reward processing and social cognition were more pronounced, while visual learning and visuo-spatial abilities were relatively preserved [14].

Beyond overdose and accidents, cardiovascular disease represents a leading cause of death among MA users. This is attributed to methamphetamine's profound effects on the cardiovascular system, including vasoconstriction, pulmonary hypertension, acceleration of atherosclerotic plaque formation, cardiac arrhythmias, and the development of cardiomyopathy [15]. The precise mechanisms underlying amphetamine-induced cardiotoxicity remain incompletely understood. However, emerging research highlights the involvement of cellular targets such as Sigma-1 receptors and trace amine-associated receptor 1 (TAAR1). Activation of these pathways triggers a cascade of adverse effects, including increased production of reactive oxygen species (ROS), mitochondrial dysfunction, and alterations in intracellular calcium homeostasis, contributing to the cardiotoxic effects of amphetamine use [16]. Methamphetamine-associated heart failure (MethHF) is an emerging clinical challenge with increasing prevalence across diverse racial, ethnic, and sociodemographic groups, predominantly affecting males. A systematic review of 21 studies revealed that up to 44% of individuals with MethHF have preserved left-ventricular ejection fraction and experience more severe heart failure symptoms compared to non-methamphetamine-related heart failure. Predictors of recovery include chamber dimensions on echocardiography, fibrosis on biopsy, female sex, MA abstinence, and adherence to guideline-directed heart failure therapy [17]. MA use and MUD have been linked to alarming increases in overdose mortality and risky patterns of use in the United States, as revealed by a cross-sectional study analyzing data from 2015 to 2019. Over this period, overdose deaths involving psychostimulants other than cocaine, largely MA, surged by 180%, while MA use increased by 43%, frequent use by 66%, and MUD without injection by 105%. The study identified the heightened prevalence of MUD among diverse populations, particularly those with lower socioeconomic status, criminal justice involvement, and comorbidities such as HIV/AIDS, hepatitis B or C, depression, and suicidal ideation. Black individuals experienced a tenfold increase in MUD prevalence, while notable rises were also observed among White, Hispanic, and LGBTQ+ populations. Risk factors for MA use and related mortality include lower educational attainment, housing instability, lack of insurance, and polysubstance use. These findings emphasize the urgent need for evidence-based prevention and treatment interventions to address the growing public health crisis associated with MA use and overdose mortality [18].

Furthermore, it imposes significant socioeconomic costs, including healthcare expenditures and loss of productivity [19–21]. The health burden of MA use in

Australia has grown significantly in recent years. Between 2010 and 2016, there was a 230% increase in demand for MA-related treatment and a 270% increase in hospital admissions due to MA-related conditions. In Queensland, the number of MA-related hospitalizations increased 20-fold between 2009 and 2015. From 2003 to 2019, treatment episodes for MA use rose more than threefold nationwide, reflecting a significant and growing need for intervention [5]. MA use among workers is notably higher than among those not in the paid workforce, with 4.0% of workers reporting use in the past 12 months compared to 2.2% of non-workers. Male workers (4.8%) reported higher MA use than female workers (3.0%), with the highest prevalence observed among 18–29-year-old workers (11.2%), particularly in industries such as hospitality (9.5%), construction (5.4%), transport (5.4%), and among tradespeople (6.5%). MA use is associated with significant workplace consequences, including higher rates of absenteeism compared to users of other illicit drugs and non-drug users. Among MA users, 13.4% reported absenteeism due to drug use, while 56.8% cited absenteeism due to any illness or injury. Additionally, 32.9% of MA users reported attending work under the influence, a significantly higher proportion than users of other illicit drugs. MA users were also more likely to engage in risky behaviors at work, such as driving, operating heavy machinery, or abusing others while under the influence, further underscoring the impact of MA use on workplace safety and productivity [22].

3. Mechanisms of methamphetamine addiction

Understanding the neurobiological underpinnings of MUD is crucial for developing effective treatments. MA exerts its effects through a multifaceted mechanism of action, primarily involving the central nervous system. It acts as a potent stimulant by increasing the release of dopamine, serotonin, and norepinephrine while simultaneously inhibiting their reuptake. MA achieves these effects through several pathways: (1) redistributing catecholamines from synaptic vesicles to the cytosol, (2) reversing plasma membrane neurotransmitter transporters, (3) inhibiting monoamine transporters, (4) reducing dopamine transporter expression on the cell surface, (5) inhibiting monoamine oxidase activity, and (6) upregulating tyrosine hydroxylase activity, the rate-limiting enzyme in dopamine synthesis. These actions result in an excessive accumulation of neurotransmitters in the synaptic cleft, leading to prolonged stimulation of postsynaptic receptors and the characteristic euphoric and stimulant effects of MA. Beyond its effects on neurotransmitter systems, MA induces significant neurotoxicity through oxidative stress, mitochondrial dysfunction, and neuroinflammation. Mitochondrial dysregulation and reactive oxygen species (ROS) production disrupt cellular homeostasis, leading to DNA damage, apoptosis, and neuronal death. MA also activates toll-like receptor 4 (TLR4) in the ventral tegmental area, further increasing dopamine release in the nucleus accumbens and contributing to neuroinflammatory cascades. This neuroinflammation, mediated by microglial activation and inflammasome pathways, exacerbates neurodegeneration and cognitive deficits [23].

The mesolimbic dopamine system, central to the brain's reward circuitry, plays a key role in MA addiction. Chronic use reduces dopamine receptor density and transporter function, requiring greater drug intake to achieve euphoric effects and diminishing the capacity for pleasure from natural rewards. Structural changes in the basal ganglia, particularly the nucleus accumbens and dorsal striatum, are linked to the reinforcement of compulsive drug-seeking behaviors and psychiatric symptoms. Additionally, MA-induced oxidative stress in the basal ganglia contributes to neurodegeneration, increasing the risk of conditions such as parkinsonism. The extended amygdala, responsible for stress and withdrawal responses, mediates the transition from seeking reward to avoiding withdrawal-related distress. This "dark side" of addiction perpetuates compulsive drug use, driven by heightened sensitivity to stress and negative reinforcement. The prefrontal cortex, critical for executive functions and impulse control, becomes increasingly impaired with prolonged MA use, leading to poor decision-making, heightened risk-taking, and reduced self-control.

Together, these disruptions in the basal ganglia, extended amygdala, and prefrontal cortex create a feedback loop that reinforces addiction. MA addiction represents a unique metabolic state characterized by oxidative stress, inflammation, and mitochondrial dysfunction, akin to mechanisms observed in neurodegenerative diseases. This neurobiological framework underscores the need for targeted interventions addressing the molecular and behavioral pathways contributing to MA addiction [24].

4. Emerging pharmacological interventions

MUD is characterized by significant neurochemical alterations, particularly within the dopaminergic system, resulting in craving, uncontrolled drug intake, and withdrawal symptoms. These disruptions arise from methamphetamine's potent effects on dopamine release, reuptake, and transporter availability, which differ significantly from those of other stimulants like cocaine. For instance, MA profoundly reduces dopamine transporter (DAT) numbers, while cocaine may increase or leave them unchanged. These distinctions, alongside the pharmacokinetic differences such as methamphetamine's longer half-life and slower clearance, underscore its more pronounced neurotoxicity and addictive potential compared to other stimulants.

MA's pharmacodynamics involve extensive dopamine dysregulation through interactions with intracellular targets, such as vesicular monoamine transporter 2 (VMAT2) and trace amine-associated receptor 1 (TAAR1). Unlike cocaine, which primarily blocks dopamine reuptake at synaptic terminals, MA facilitates dopamine release and reduces intracellular degradation, leading to excessive synaptic dopamine accumulation. This dopamine surge not only drives euphoria and reinforcement but also contributes to oxidative stress, neuroinflammation, and structural brain damage. These mechanisms highlight the need for pharmacological treatments targeting dopamine pathways to restore neurochemical balance and mitigate addiction-related behaviors [25].

4.1 Dopaminergic agents

Dopaminergic drugs represent a key area of research and development in pharmacotherapy for MUD due to their ability to modulate dopamine signaling, a central mechanism in MUD. The following summarizes their rational mechanisms and clinical efficacy:

4.1.1 Psychostimulants

Psychostimulants such as lisdexamfetamine (LDX), dextroamphetamine (AMPH), and methylphenidate (MPH), primarily used for attention-deficit/hyperactivity disorder (ADHD), act by enhancing the release of dopamine and norepinephrine into synapses. AMPH also inhibits vesicular monoamine transporter-2 (VMAT-2) function and monoamine oxidase (MAO) activity, while MPH inhibits dopamine and norepinephrine reuptake. In the context of MUD, these drugs have been explored as substitution therapies to reduce the harm associated with MA use by providing a safer alternative to illicit drug administration. While AMPH blunts some subjective effects of MA, preclinical studies have shown limited efficacy, and MPH may even potentiate MA's reinforcing effects. Furthermore, both drugs carry risks of misuse and diversion, highlighting the need for cautious clinical use [26]. A systematic review of 43 randomized controlled trials encompassing 4065 participants evaluated 23 pharmacological treatments for MUD. While no pharmacotherapy demonstrated consistently robust efficacy, stimulant agonist treatments (dexamphetamine and methylphenidate), naltrexone, and topiramate showed the most promising results. Some antidepressants like bupropion and mirtazapine and agents such as riluzole and pexacerfont showed less consistent benefits, whereas SSRIs and TCAs were largely ineffective. Many studies were underpowered with low treatment completion rates, highlighting the need for larger trials with standardized outcome measures, such as changes in use days [27]. A randomized, double-blind, placebo-controlled trial in Australia (2018–2021) evaluated the efficacy and safety of a 12-week lisdexamfetamine regimen for reducing MA use among 164 adults with MA dependence. While benefits at week 13 were minimal (adjusted difference = 2.2 days, 95% CI = −0.5 to 5.0; $P = 0.49$), lisdexamfetamine significantly reduced MA use over the entire treatment period (difference = 8.8 days, 95% CI = 2.7–15.0; $P = 0.005$) and improved treatment satisfaction (OR = 3.80, 95% CI = 1.93–7.47; $P < 0.001$). Adverse events, including nausea, were reported in 5% of participants. These results suggest lisdexamfetamine may effectively reduce MA use during the treatment period [28].

4.1.2 Atomoxetine

Atomoxetine, a selective norepinephrine transporter inhibitor, represents a non-stimulant alternative to traditional psychostimulants. Atomoxetine shows potential as a treatment for MUD in individuals on methadone maintenance therapy (MMT). In a double-blind, placebo-controlled trial with 86 participants, those receiving atomoxetine (40 mg/day) showed significant reductions in MA craving ($P < 0.001$) and higher rates of negative MA urine tests (56% vs. 26%, $P = 0.007$) after 8 weeks. Atomoxetine also reduced depression, anxiety, and stress more effectively than placebo ($P < 0.05$ for all). The treatment was well-tolerated with mild side effects, supporting its safety and potential efficacy in managing MUD [29]. In a double-blind, placebo-controlled trial involving 69 male participants (mean age 39.4 years), those receiving atomoxetine (80 mg daily) had a higher proportion of ATS-negative urine tests compared to placebo: 0.77 vs. 0.67 ($d = 0.26$) in the intention-to-treat (ITT) sample and 0.90 vs. 0.64 ($d = 0.56$) among participants with higher adherence (≥60 days of treatment). Both groups showed increased days of ATS abstinence and reduced depressive symptoms, with greater improvement in the atomoxetine group ($P < 0.02$). Atomoxetine was well-tolerated, with no serious adverse events or discontinuations due to side effects, supporting its safety and potential use in this population [30].

4.1.3 Modafinil

Modafinil, a weak dopamine transporter inhibitor, demonstrates neuroprotective effects, including reduced MA-induced neuroinflammation, dopamine toxicity, and neuronal death. A randomized, double-blind, placebo-controlled study assessed modafinil's efficacy in reducing MA use among 210 participants with DSM-IV MA dependence. Participants received placebo (n = 68), modafinil 200 mg (n = 72), or modafinil 400 mg (n = 70) daily for 12 weeks, with thrice-weekly clinic visits for assessments, urine drug screens, and group psychotherapy. The primary outcome, MA non-use weeks, showed no significant difference between modafinil and placebo groups (P = 0.53). Secondary outcomes were also not significant. However, an ad-hoc analysis revealed participants with high medication compliance (>85% confirmed by urinalysis) had a longer maximum duration of abstinence (23 days vs. 10 days, P = 0.003). While modafinil was not conclusively effective, results may be limited by inadequate medication adherence [31].

4.1.4 Bupropion

Bupropion, a norepinephrine-dopamine reuptake inhibitor and VMAT-2 modulator, has shown promise in preclinical models by reducing MA self-administration and blunting positive subjective effects of the drug. A double-blind, placebo-controlled study evaluated bupropion's efficacy in increasing abstinence weeks among 151 participants with DSM-IV MA dependence. Participants received sustained-release bupropion 150 mg twice daily (n = 79) or placebo (n = 72) for 12 weeks, with thrice-weekly clinic visits for assessments, urine drug screens, and group therapy. While overall differences in MA-free weeks between groups were not statistically significant (P = 0.09), subgroup analysis revealed a significant benefit for bupropion among male participants with lower baseline MA use (P < 0.0001). Comorbid conditions such as depression and ADHD did not affect outcomes, suggesting bupropion's potential efficacy in low-to-moderate dependence, particularly in males [32]. Bupropion also shows benefits in comorbid PTSD and MUD, as evidenced by a case series comparing it to serotonergic agents. Patients receiving bupropion experienced greater reductions in PTSD checklist-civilian scores (77 to 35 to 29) versus those on serotonergic agents (51 ± 15 to 52 ± 20 to 53 ± 10). Bupropion users also had lower relapse rates (25.0% vs. 48.8%), longer time to relapse (107 vs. 210 ± 191 days), and no hospitalizations (0% vs. 29.3%). These findings suggest bupropion may effectively address PTSD symptoms and reduce MA relapse in this population [33].

4.1.5 VMAT-2 inhibitors

VMAT-2 inhibitors, such as lobeline and its analogs, target dopamine storage and release mechanisms. Preclinical studies demonstrate significant reductions in MA self-administration, cue-induced reinstatement, and conditioned place preference (CPP) without tolerance development. Although human studies are lacking, these findings suggest that VMAT-2 inhibitors could be a promising direction for MUD pharmacotherapy [26].

4.1.6 Antipsychotics

Antipsychotics play a critical role in managing methamphetamine psychosis (MAP), as demonstrated by a network meta-analysis (NMA) of six randomized controlled trials (RCTs) including 395 MAP patients. The study evaluated six antipsychotics: aripiprazole, haloperidol, olanzapine, paliperidone extended-release, quetiapine, and risperidone. Olanzapine and quetiapine were found to be more effective than risperidone, while aripiprazole showed lower efficacy compared to olanzapine, quetiapine, haloperidol, and paliperidone. Dropout rates were similar across treatments. These findings suggest that certain antipsychotics, such as olanzapine and quetiapine, may offer superior benefits in MAP treatment. This rationale supports exploring antipsychotics' potential in managing MUD by addressing associated psychosis and behavioral disturbances [34]. A retrospective chart review evaluated the efficacy and safety of aripiprazole in maintaining abstinence among Thai patients with MA dependence following MA psychosis. Forty-three patients (aged 18–65 years) received aripiprazole (2.5–15 mg/day) for at least 2 weeks post-psychosis resolution. Abstinence rates, assessed by urine toxicology, were 90.7% at week 2 and 75% at week 12. Common adverse events included parkinsonism (11.63%), insomnia (6.98%), sedation (6.98%), and akathisia (4.65%). Aripiprazole showed efficacy in maintaining abstinence and was generally safe and well-tolerated in this population [35]. Aripiprazole has been investigated as a potential treatment for MUD, a significant public health issue lacking FDA- or EMA-approved pharmacotherapies. A systematic review and meta-analysis examined the efficacy of various pharmacological agents, including antidepressants, antipsychotics, psychostimulants, anticonvulsants, and opioid antagonists, across 17 randomized controlled trials (RCTs) involving sample sizes ranging from 19 to 229 participants. For aripiprazole specifically, the evidence was of low strength and suggested no significant effect on key outcomes such as abstinence, as defined by three or more consecutive weeks with negative urine drug screens (UDS), or on overall MA/A use and treatment retention [36].

Dopaminergic drugs for MUD provide diverse mechanisms for addressing dopamine dysregulation. Substitution therapies (e.g., AMPH and MPH) aim to reduce harm but require careful management due to misuse potential. Alternatives like atomoxetine and modafinil offer additional benefits, including reduced cravings and neuroprotection, while drugs targeting VMAT-2 represent an innovative approach in preclinical research. Combining these pharmacotherapies with behavioral interventions could enhance treatment outcomes, although further studies are needed to optimize efficacy and mitigate risks [26].

4.2 Glutamatergic modulators

Medications such as N-acetylcysteine (NAC) target the glutamate system, aiming to restore the neurochemical balance disrupted by MA use. Preliminary studies indicate reductions in cravings and improvements in cognitive function. In a double-blind, randomized, placebo-controlled trial. Participants (N = 153) were assigned to receive NAC (2400 mg/day) or placebo for 12 weeks. MA use, assessed *via* Timeline Follow back and MA-positive oral fluid samples, showed significant reduction in both groups but no additional benefit of NAC over placebo. Secondary outcomes, including craving, dependence severity, withdrawal symptoms, and psychiatric symptoms, also showed no significant differences between groups. Adverse events were comparable, suggesting NAC was well-tolerated but ineffective in reducing MA use or improving related clinical outcomes [37].

Topiramate has shown potential as a pharmacotherapy targeting the glutamatergic system for managing MUD. A double-blind, placebo-controlled trial evaluated its efficacy for MUD in 140 adults randomized to topiramate (up to 200 mg/day) or placebo for 13 weeks, alongside behavioral therapy. While topiramate did not significantly increase abstinence during weeks 6–12, it reduced MA levels and dependence severity. Participants abstinent before randomization demonstrated greater abstinence on topiramate compared to placebo [38]. A randomized, double-blind, placebo-controlled clinical trial evaluated its effectiveness in 52 patients aged 16–60 years, divided into an intervention group (n = 26) receiving topiramate (50 mg titrated to 200 mg daily) and a placebo group (n = 26). Over 12 weeks, participants were assessed using the Beck Depression Inventory, a drug use temptation questionnaire, urine tests, and a side effects questionnaire. While no significant differences were observed in depression scores or urine test results across the groups, the intervention group demonstrated significantly reduced drug craving compared to placebo in the 8th, 10th, and 12th weeks ($P < 0.05$). These findings suggest topiramate may reduce craving in MUD patients, though additional studies are required to confirm these outcomes [39].

4.3 Immunotherapy approaches

MA vaccines and monoclonal antibodies are novel strategies aimed at reducing the psychoactive effects of the drug by preventing its entry into the central nervous system. Recent advances focus on active vaccination strategies, such as hapten design, and passive immunization with monoclonal antibodies. Preclinical studies have demonstrated progress, though clinical evaluation remains limited [40]. Recent progress includes the development of a novel conjugated vaccine using MA HCl as a hapten, a peptide linker composed of lysine and glycine, and an immunogenic carrier, oxidized mannan (OM). Analytical techniques confirmed successful chemical conjugation, and the vaccine demonstrated stability under various storage conditions for 3 months. Animal studies further supported its immunogenicity, producing a robust antibody response. These findings provide a foundation for future preclinical studies to evaluate the vaccine's potential in preventing MA addiction [41]. Two vaccines, IXTv-100 with adjuvant GLA-SE and TT-SMA with alum and adjuvant E6020, have shown efficacy in reducing MA-induced behaviors by generating robust antibody responses. These vaccine behavior and TH levels in the brain, attenuate drug-seeking behavior, and mitigate MA's effects on the reward system. Both approaches were well-tolerated in rodent studies, demonstrating potential for further research. However, clinical trials remain limited, and challenges such as ensuring adherence and addressing psychological dependence must be addressed to advance these vaccines for human use [24].

Immunotherapy offers a promising avenue for addressing MUD by targeting neuroimmune signaling, which plays a critical role in the neurobiology of addiction. Psychoactive substances like MA can alter glial cell activity, microglial activation markers, and cytokine levels, contributing to neuroinflammation and behavioral changes associated with addiction. Immunomodulators such as minocycline and ibudilast have shown potential in preclinical and clinical studies. Minocycline, a microglial inhibitor, reverses MA-induced behavioral and neurochemical alterations and improves psychotic symptoms, while ibudilast reduces MA craving and reward-related effects, with anti-inflammatory properties being a key mechanism. These drugs are well-tolerated with minimal side effects, making them viable candidates for further exploration. Understanding how glial and neuroinflammatory responses influence addiction may guide the development of novel therapeutic strategies for substance use disorders, including MUD [42].

5. Behavioral or psychological interventions

Behavioral and psychological interventions are the cornerstone of treatment for MUD, providing evidence-based strategies to reduce drug use, manage cravings, and support recovery. These interventions target the underlying behavioral and cognitive patterns associated with MUD, emphasizing skills development, motivation enhancement, and lifestyle changes. Key approaches include:

5.1 Cognitive-behavioral therapy (CBT)

CBT focuses on identifying and changing maladaptive thought patterns and behaviors related to drug use. It equips patients with coping strategies to manage triggers, stress, and cravings, demonstrating efficacy both as a standalone treatment and when combined with other interventions.

CBT remains a cornerstone of MUD treatment, focusing on modifying maladaptive thoughts and behaviors. Psychological interventions, particularly cognitive-behavioral therapy (CBT) and contingency management (CM), have proven effective in addressing MA use and dependence, especially given the limited efficacy of pharmacological treatments. A systematic review of randomized trials found that CBT consistently reduced MA use and achieved positive outcomes, even with brief interventions of 2–4 sessions. CM demonstrated significant reductions in MA use during treatment, though its long-term effects post-treatment remain uncertain. These interventions are accessible and can be seamlessly integrated into alcohol and other drug (AOD) services. AOD clinicians should adopt and advocate for these evidence-based approaches, while further research is needed to enhance the longevity of their effects and improve outcomes for more complex cases [43]. A systematic review of 44 studies evaluated non-pharmaceutical approaches for MUD, identifying effective behavioral interventions such as cognitive-behavioral therapy (CBT), contingency management (CM), exercise, residential rehabilitation, repetitive transcranial magnetic stimulation (rTMS), and the Matrix Model. Among these, CM demonstrated the strongest evidence for promoting abstinence, reducing MA use, and decreasing cravings, while tailored CBT, either alone or combined with CM, was also effective. Behavioral interventions should be prioritized as first-line treatments for MUD, with future research needed to address the sustainability of effects, small sample sizes, and high dropout rates [44].

A systematic review of randomized controlled trials assessed the effectiveness of psychological interventions on both MA use and psychiatric symptom outcomes. Utilizing Cochrane and PRISMA guidelines, 10 eligible studies were reviewed. Most studies reported reductions in MA use and psychiatric symptoms, with evidence suggesting that more intensive interventions yielded greater benefits compared to brief approaches. Attendance rates varied across studies. Overall, psychological treatments effectively reduced MA use and improved psychiatric symptoms, highlighting the need for future research to optimize outcomes in both domains and enhance treatment adherence [45].

Innovations in delivery, such as digital CBT, have expanded access and engagement. A digital cognitive-behavioral therapy (CBT) program, Breaking Free from Substance Abuse, was introduced in May 2020 to address MA use among 2187 incarcerated individuals in Ohio prisons, marking its first widespread use in U.S. correctional facilities. Participants reported significant psychosocial risk factors, including substance dependence, mental health issues, interpersonal conflict, and socioeconomic challenges. The program demonstrated significant reductions in substance dependence, depression/anxiety, and biopsychosocial impairment, alongside improved quality of life. Positive outcomes were linked to program engagement and completion of specific components, with a dose-response effect observed. Digital

CBT offers a viable treatment option in correctional settings, helping address MA use among incarcerated individuals while mitigating barriers to in-person therapy [46]. Echo-APP, a tablet-based digital psychotherapist app, was developed to address inequities in access to substance use disorder (SUD) treatment and piloted in 47 patients with MUD. The app includes assessment tools for mood, impulsivity, craving, and motivation, along with 10 treatment units focusing on addiction awareness, motivation enhancement, and emotion regulation. After a single session, participants showed significant improvements in treatment motivation and drug abstinence confidence, alongside reduced cravings. Predictive factors included baseline anxiety and impulsivity scores. These findings demonstrate Echo-APP's feasibility and potential as a remote therapeutic tool for MUD, warranting further large-scale studies [47].

5.2 Contingency management (CM)

CM employs positive reinforcement, such as vouchers or incentives, to reward abstinence and adherence to treatment. This approach has shown robust results in promoting sustained abstinence in MUD patients. A systematic review encompassing 27 studies, including 10 new randomized controlled trials, highlights CM's efficacy in diverse populations, including men who have sex with men (MSM), general community settings, and research treatment programs. CM has demonstrated broad benefits, including increased drug abstinence, higher utilization of medical and treatment services, and reduced risky sexual behaviors. Of the studies reporting abstinence outcomes, 20 out of 21 showed significant effects of CM, and seven of nine studies reporting sexual risk behavior outcomes demonstrated reductions in risky behaviors. These findings underscore the importance of prioritizing CM in outpatient programs for MUD as a highly effective, evidence-based treatment strategy [48].

5.3 Mindfulness-based interventions

Mindfulness practices, such as mindfulness-based relapse prevention, address the psychological components of addiction, including stress and emotional dysregulation. Mindfulness-based interventions (MBIs) have emerged as promising treatments for MA addiction. Recent studies indicate that MBIs can significantly reduce cravings, decrease relapse risks, and alleviate stress, depression, and aggression in individuals with MUD. Notably, combining mindfulness practices with transcranial direct current stimulation (tDCS) has shown enhanced efficacy in improving cognitive functions among MA users. The therapeutic effects of mindfulness may be attributed to its potential to induce neuroplastic changes, thereby mitigating addiction symptoms. However, further high-quality research, incorporating neuroimaging and neurophysiological measures, is essential to fully understand the mechanisms underlying mindfulness in treating MA addiction and to establish its role as a standard treatment option [49].

5.4 Exercise-based interventions

Physical activity has shown promise in reducing cravings, improving mood, and promoting overall well-being, making it a valuable complement to traditional therapies. An 8-week structured exercise intervention was evaluated for its efficacy in reducing MA use among 135 individuals following residential treatment. Participants were randomized into an exercise group or a health education control group, with follow-up assessments at 1, 3, and 6 months post-discharge. While overall differences between groups in returning to MA use were not statistically significant, a significant interaction was observed for lower severity users (using MA ≤18 days in the month before admission). Those in the exercise group reported fewer days of MA use and had lower rates of positive urine tests compared to their counterparts in the education group at all follow-up points. No significant differences were found for higher-severity users. These findings suggest that structured exercise may benefit individuals with lower baseline severity of MA use [50]. A systematic review evaluated the effects of physical activity on negative emotions, cognitive impairment, and drug craving in individuals with MUD. Seventeen studies, encompassing 1836 participants, were included, focusing on interventions using clearly defined physical activity and reporting measurable outcomes in mood, cognition, and craving. Results indicate that physical activity-based interventions can effectively manage withdrawal symptoms and improve drug rehabilitation outcomes by alleviating negative emotions, enhancing cognitive function, and reducing drug cravings [51].

5.5 The matrix model

This structured, multi-component program integrates individual therapy, group therapy, and family education, focusing on relapse prevention, motivation enhancement, and lifestyle changes. It is particularly effective in outpatient settings for individuals with MUD. The Matrix Model, combined with methylphenidate (MPH), has demonstrated significant therapeutic benefits for people who use methamphetamine (PWUM). A clinical trial involving 100 participants evaluated the effects of 12 weeks of treatment across four groups: Matrix Model alone, MPH alone, Matrix Model with MPH, and a control group. Results showed that the combination of Matrix Model treatment with MPH significantly reduced MA craving and addiction severity while improving mental health compared to the other groups ($P < 0.001$). Additionally, participants in the combined treatment group had higher rates of negative MA urine tests ($P < 0.001$). These findings suggest that integrating MPH with the Matrix Model enhances outcomes for addiction severity, craving, relapse prevention, and mental health in PWUM [52].

5.6 Residential rehabilitation-based therapies

Residential rehabilitation-based therapies provide structured, intensive treatment for individuals with MUD in a supportive, drug-free environment. These programs typically combine behavioral therapies, such as cognitive-behavioral therapy (CBT) and contingency management (CM), with skills training, group counseling, and relapse prevention strategies. Studies indicate that residential rehabilitation reduces craving and psychiatric symptoms, while improving psychosocial resources, processing speed, and cognitive flexibility. However, no significant differences were observed in treatment completion rates or outcomes between the two approaches. A high dropout rate (40.7%) was noted, with a history of injection drug use predicting a higher dropout risk [53]. The study in long-term was conducted in Germany. Among 108 participants, follow-ups at 12 months (T2) and 18 months (T3) showed MA abstinence rates of 77.1% and 68.0%, respectively, among those who completed follow-ups. When assuming relapse for non-follow-up participants, abstinence rates were 25.0% (T2) and 15.7% (T3). No significant differences in MA use were observed between treatment programs or between completers and dropouts. Injection drug use predicted MA use at T2, and higher depression scores at T2 predicted MA use at T3. Dropouts at T2 reported higher craving scores than completers. Median relapse occurred 1.5 days post-discharge. These findings highlight the positive effects of residential treatments but emphasize the need to improve transitions to outpatient care and address treatment dropout. Further research is needed to explore these factors and reduce study attrition [54].

6. Neurostimulation techniques

Neurostimulation techniques, including repetitive transcranial magnetic stimulation (rTMS), transcranial direct current stimulation (tDCS), and deep brain stimulation (DBS), have emerged as promising interventions for MUD. These non-invasive or minimally invasive methods aim to modulate brain activity in regions implicated in addiction, such as the prefrontal cortex, striatum, and limbic system, which are involved in reward processing, impulse control, and craving regulation.

6.1 Repetitive transcranial magnetic stimulation (rTMS)

rTMS applies electromagnetic pulses to stimulate neuronal activity, often targeting the dorsolateral prefrontal cortex (DLPFC). Studies have shown that rTMS can reduce craving and improve cognitive control in individuals with MUD by enhancing prefrontal activity and mitigating the overactivation of the mesolimbic reward pathway. Sessions are typically short and well-tolerated, making rTMS a feasible outpatient treatment. A systematic review and meta-analysis of seven double-blind, randomized controlled trials involving 462 participants revealed that rTMS significantly reduced craving scores compared to sham treatments ($SMD = 0.983$, $CI = 0.620–1.345$, $P \leq 0.001$). Among the rTMS protocols, intermittent theta-burst stimulation (iTBS) demonstrated greater efficacy in craving reduction than standard 10-Hz rTMS. A metaregression analysis further indicated that higher baseline craving scores were associated with greater treatment effects, whereas higher proportions of male participants and longer durations of abstinence were linked to diminished efficacy. These findings highlight the therapeutic potential of rTMS, particularly iTBS, as an adjunctive treatment for reducing cravings in MUD, warranting further investigation into its optimization and broader clinical application [55].

6.2 Transcranial direct current stimulation (tDCS)

tDCS delivers low-intensity electrical currents to modulate cortical excitability. It has shown potential in reducing drug craving and improving executive function in MUD patients. By stimulating the DLPFC, tDCS aims to restore the balance between cognitive control and reward-related impulsivity, often disrupted in MUD. A quasi-experimental study examined the effects of transcranial direct current stimulation (tDCS) across six stimulation protocols on reducing drug craving and enhancing cognitive inhibition in 15 male MA addicts. Participants underwent pre- and post-assessments, including the Visual Analog Scale (VAS), go/no-go task, and n-back task, before and after a single tDCS session. Results showed that while single-session tDCS did not significantly reduce craving, it notably increased cognitive inhibition, particularly in the protocol involving right DLPFC cathodal and left DLPFC anodal stimulation. These findings highlight the potential of tDCS to improve cognitive control in addiction recovery, suggesting its value as a non-invasive intervention to enhance inhibitory control, even if immediate craving reduction remains limited [56].

6.3 Deep brain stimulation (DBS)

DBS involves the implantation of electrodes to modulate neural circuits associated with addiction. While primarily experimental, early studies demonstrate promise for treatment-resistant MUD. A study using an MA-conditioned place preference (CPP) paradigm in rats evaluated the effects of high-frequency (HFS: 130 Hz) and low-frequency stimulation (LFS: 13 Hz) applied during either the conditioning or extinction phases of MA-induced CPP. Results demonstrated that both HFS and LFS significantly reduced MA place preference during the conditioning phase, while HFS during the extinction phase accelerated the extinction of reward-context associations and reduced reinstatement of drug-seeking behavior. These findings highlight the potential of DBS in the OFC to suppress the development, maintenance, and relapse of MA-seeking behaviors, supporting further preclinical exploration of DBS as a treatment modality for psychostimulant use disorders [57].

Although neurostimulation offers a novel approach to treating MUD, challenges remain. Limited large-scale trials, variability in treatment protocols, and the need for long-term outcome data hinder widespread adoption. Future research should focus on optimizing stimulation parameters, identifying patient subgroups most likely to benefit, and integrating neurostimulation with behavioral therapies for comprehensive care.

In summary, neurostimulation techniques represent an innovative and potentially transformative avenue for MUD treatment. They offer a non-pharmacological approach to addressing the neurobiological underpinnings of addiction, with the potential to enhance recovery and reduce relapse rates. Continued research is crucial to establish their role in routine clinical practice.

7. Future directions

Future treatments for MUD should prioritize the integration of multimodal therapies, combining pharmacological, behavioral, and neurostimulation approaches to maximize therapeutic outcomes. Pharmacological interventions targeting neurotransmitter imbalances, when paired with evidence-based behavioral therapies like contingency management (CM) or cognitive-behavioral therapy (CBT), could enhance adherence and address the psychological aspects of addiction. Additionally, emerging neurostimulation techniques, such as transcranial magnetic stimulation (TMS) and deep brain stimulation (DBS), show promise in modulating brain circuits involved in craving and reward processing. A synergistic approach that incorporates these modalities has the potential to address the complex neurobiological and psychological dimensions of MUD, offering patients a comprehensive and individualized pathway to recovery.

Real-time monitoring and intervention could enhance treatment efficacy beyond conventional methods like behavioral therapy and peer support. An intelligent closed-loop transcranial magnetic stimulation (TMS) neuromodulation system using multimodal electroencephalogram-functional near-infrared spectroscopy (EEG-fNIRS) offers a promising solution. This system leverages neuroimaging's advantages over traditional biomarkers (e.g., sweat, saliva, and urine) for addiction detection.

Key EEG biomarkers include frequency, time-domain, and topography-related parameters, while fNIRS focuses on hemoglobin concentration and cortical connectivity. The integration of EEG-fNIRS with neuromodulation techniques like TMS and transcranial direct current stimulation (tDCS) could provide targeted, user-friendly interventions for MUD. Challenges remain in implementing wearable, compact, closed-loop systems, but this approach holds promise for transforming addiction treatment and extending applications to other substance use disorders [58].

Advances in neuroimaging, specifically high-density electroencephalography (EEG), have demonstrated promise in identifying individual-level neurobiological signatures of craving. By analyzing beta-band functional connectivity during resting states, researchers have developed predictive models that differentiate individuals with MUD from healthy controls and accurately gauge craving intensity. These findings highlight the potential of EEG-based connectome models to guide personalized treatment strategies for MUD. By dissecting neurophysiological features, such models offer a pathway to tailored interventions that address the unique neurobiological underpinnings of craving, improving outcomes and reducing relapse risk [59].

Epigenetic mechanisms in MUD such as DNA methylation, histone modifications, and non-coding RNA activity, which dysregulate gene expression in neuroreward pathways, altering brain function and structure. Advanced technologies like high-throughput sequencing and RNA sequencing have identified specific epigenetic markers linked to MA addiction, providing potential therapeutic targets. By reversing these epigenetic changes, novel treatments could mitigate neurotoxicity and improve addiction recovery. Future research should focus on translating these findings into personalized therapies that modulate epigenetic mechanisms, offering a promising path for more effective management of MUD [60].

8. Conclusions

MUD remains a significant global public health challenge, driven by the drug's potent addictive properties and its widespread availability. This chapter has explored various facets of MUD, including its neurobiological underpinnings, psychological and behavioral interventions, and emerging treatment modalities. Current research highlights the complexity of MUD, emphasizing the need for integrative approaches that combine pharmacological, behavioral, and neuromodulation therapies to address both the addiction itself and its associated psychiatric comorbidities.

Advancements in neuroimaging, epigenetics, and biomarkers offer promising avenues for developing personalized treatments, enabling better prediction of treatment response and relapse risk. Moreover, innovative technologies such as wearable closed-loop neuromodulation systems hold potential for real-time intervention and relapse prevention. Despite progress, challenges remain in translating preclinical findings into effective clinical applications, necessitating further research and larger-scale trials.

Future trends in MUD treatment underscore the importance of addressing stigma, increasing accessibility to evidence-based interventions, and fostering collaborations between healthcare providers, researchers, and policymakers. By building on the insights presented in this chapter, the development of more effective, sustainable, and personalized strategies for MUD management is achievable, offering hope to individuals and communities affected by this pervasive disorder.

Acknowledgements

The author extends heartfelt gratitude to Associate Professor Dr. Thanarat Suansane, Faculty of Pharmacy, Mahidol University, Thailand for providing invaluable expertise and guidance in the management of patients with substance use disorders and for his significant contributions to the research project on MA conducted at the Princess Mother National Institute of Drug Abuse Treatment in Thailand.

Conflict of interest

The author declares no conflict of interest.

Author details

Tuanthon Boonlue
Faculty of Pharmaceutical Sciences, Ubon Ratchathani University, Ubon Ratchathani, Thailand

*Address all correspondence to: tuanthon.b@ubu.ac.th

References

[1] Ballester J, Marchand WR, Philip NS. Transcranial magnetic stimulation for methamphetamine use disorder: A scoping review within the neurocircuitry model of addiction. Psychiatry Research. 2024;**338**:115995. DOI: 10.1016/j.psychres.2024.115995

[2] Moszczynska A. Current and emerging treatments for methamphetamine use disorder. Current Neuropharmacology. 2021;**19**(12):2077-2091. DOI: 10.2174/1570159x19666210803091637

[3] United Nations Office on Drugs and Crime. World Drug Report 2024. United Nations Publication; 2024

[4] Jones CM, Houry D, Han B, Baldwin G, Vivolo-Kantor A, Compton WM. Methamphetamine use in the United States: Epidemiological update and implications for prevention, treatment, and harm reduction. Annals of the New York Academy of Sciences. 2022;**1508**(1):3-22. DOI: 10.1111/nyas.14688

[5] Scott R. Methamphetamine dependence in Australia-why is 'ice' (crystal meth) so addictive? Psychiatry, Psychology and Law. 2024;**31**(4):671-704. DOI: 10.1080/13218719.2023.2206870

[6] The Lancet Regional Health-Southeast Asia. Escape from quicksand: Illicit drug use among youth in southeast Asia. The Lancet Regional Health – Southeast Asia. 2023;**10**:100175. DOI: 10.1016/j.lansea.2023.100175

[7] Hançer Tok H, Tokur KM. Reasons for using methamphetamine: Systematic review. Archives of Psychiatric Nursing. 2024;**52**:147-154. DOI: 10.1016/j.apnu.2024.07.007

[8] Rastegari A, Haghdoost AA, Baneshi MR, Azizian M, Mehrolhassani MH. Identifying the factors affecting methamphetamine use: A scoping review. Medical Journal of the Islamic Republic of Iran. 2023;**37**:102. DOI: 10.47176/mjiri.37.102

[9] Marshall BD, Werb D. Health outcomes associated with methamphetamine use among young people: A systematic review. Addiction. 2010;**105**(6):991-1002. DOI: 10.1111/j.1360-0443.2010.02932.x

[10] Guerin AA, Bridson T, Plapp HM, Bedi G. A systematic review and meta-analysis of health, functional, and cognitive outcomes in young people who use methamphetamine. Neuroscience and Biobehavioral Reviews. 2023;**153**:105380. DOI: 10.1016/j.neubiorev.2023.105380

[11] Leung J, Mekonen T, Wang X, Arunogiri S, Degenhardt L, McKetin R. Methamphetamine exposure and depression—A systematic review and meta-analysis. Drug and Alcohol Review. 2023;**42**(6):1438-1449. DOI: 10.1111/dar.13670

[12] Cohen-Laroque J, Grangier I, Perez N, Kirschner M, Kaiser S, Sabé M. Positive and negative symptoms in methamphetamine-induced psychosis compared to schizophrenia: A systematic review and meta-analysis. Schizophrenia Research. 2024;**267**:182-190. DOI: 10.1016/j.schres.2024.03.037

[13] McKetin R, Leung J, Stockings E, Huo Y, Foulds J, Lappin JM, et al. Mental health outcomes associated with of the use of amphetamines: A systematic review and meta-analysis. EClinicalMedicine. 2019;**16**:81-97. DOI: 10.1016/j.eclinm.2019.09.014

[14] Potvin S, Pelletier J, Grot S, Hébert C, Barr AM, Lecomte T. Cognitive deficits in individuals with methamphetamine use disorder: A meta-analysis. Addictive Behaviors. 2018;**80**:154-160. DOI: 10.1016/j.addbeh.2018.01.021

[15] Kevil CG, Goeders NE, Woolard MD, Bhuiyan MS, Dominic P, Kolluru GK, et al. Methamphetamine use and cardiovascular disease. Arteriosclerosis, Thrombosis, and Vascular Biology. 2019;**39**(9):1739-1746. DOI: 10.1161/atvbaha.119.312461

[16] Tobolski J, Sawyer DB, Song SJ, Afari ME. Cardiovascular disease associated with methamphetamine use: A review. Heart Failure Reviews. 2022;**27**(6):2059-2065. DOI: 10.1007/s10741-022-10261-7

[17] Manja V, Nrusimha A, Gao Y, Sheikh A, McGovern M, Heidenreich PA, et al. Methamphetamine-associated heart failure: A systematic review of observational studies. Heart. 2023;**109**(3):168-177. DOI: 10.1136/heartjnl-2022-321610

[18] Han B, Compton WM, Jones CM, Einstein EB, Volkow ND. Methamphetamine use, methamphetamine use disorder, and associated overdose deaths among US adults. JAMA Psychiatry. 2021;**78**(12):1329-1342. DOI: 10.1001/jamapsychiatry.2021.2588

[19] Zhao SX, Deluna A, Kelsey K, Wang C, Swaminathan A, Staniec A, et al. Socioeconomic burden of rising methamphetamine-associated heart failure hospitalizations in California from 2008 to 2018. Circulation. Cardiovascular Quality and Outcomes. 2021;**14**(7):e007638. DOI: 10.1161/circoutcomes.120.007638

[20] Tait RJ, Whetton S, Shanahan M, Cartwright K, Ferrante A, Gray D, et al. Quantifying the societal cost of methamphetamine use to Australia. The International Journal on Drug Policy. 2018;**62**:30-36. DOI: 10.1016/j.drugpo.2018.08.015

[21] Reddy P, Elkayam U. The hidden cost of meth: Appraising the socioeconomic burden of methamphetamine-associated cardiomyopathy. Circulation. Cardiovascular Quality and Outcomes. 2021;**14**(7):e008214. DOI: 10.1161/circoutcomes.121.008214

[22] Roche AM, Pidd K, Bywood P, Freeman T. Methamphetamine use among Australian workers and its implications for prevention. Drug and Alcohol Review. 2008;**27**(3):334-341. DOI: 10.1080/09595230801919478

[23] Paulus MP, Stewart JL. Neurobiology, clinical presentation, and treatment of methamphetamine use disorder: A review. JAMA Psychiatry. 2020;**77**(9):959-966. DOI: 10.1001/jamapsychiatry.2020.0246

[24] Prasad S, Mathew PS, Piper BJ, Kaur K, Tian M. The neurobiology of methamphetamine addiction and the potential to reduce misuse through conjugate vaccines targeting toll-like receptor 4. Cureus. 2023;**15**(6):e40259. DOI: 10.7759/cureus.40259

[25] Kohno M, Dennis LE, McCready H, Hoffman WF. Dopamine dysfunction in stimulant use disorders: Mechanistic comparisons and implications for treatment. Molecular Psychiatry. 2022;**27**(1):220-229. DOI: 10.1038/s41380-021-01180-4

[26] Yates JR. Pharmacological treatments for methamphetamine use disorder: Current status and future targets. Substance Abuse and Rehabilitation. 2024;**15**:125-161. DOI: 10.2147/sar.S431273

[27] Siefried KJ, Acheson LS, Lintzeris N, Ezard N. Pharmacological treatment of methamphetamine/amphetamine dependence: A systematic review. CNS Drugs. 2020;**34**(4):337-365. DOI: 10.1007/s40263-020-00711-x

[28] Ezard N, Clifford B, Siefried KJ, Ali R, Dunlop A, McKetin R, et al. Lisdexamfetamine in the treatment of methamphetamine dependence: A randomised, placebo-controlled trial. Addiction. 2024. DOI: 10.1111/add.16730 [Online ahead of print]

[29] Rabiey A, Hassani-Abharian P, Farhad M, Moravveji AR, Akasheh G, Banafshe HR. Atomoxetine efficacy in methamphetamine dependence during methadone maintenance therapy. Archives of Iranian Medicine. 2019;**22**(12):692-698

[30] Schottenfeld RS, Chawarski MC, Sofuoglu M, Chooi WT, Zaharim NM, Yasin MAM, et al. Atomoxetine for amphetamine-type stimulant dependence during buprenorphine treatment: A randomized controlled trial. Drug and Alcohol Dependence. 2018;**186**:130-137. DOI: 10.1016/j.drugalcdep.2018.01.017

[31] Anderson AL, Li SH, Biswas K, McSherry F, Holmes T, Iturriaga E, et al. Modafinil for the treatment of methamphetamine dependence. Drug and Alcohol Dependence. 2012;**120**(1-3):135-141. DOI: 10.1016/j.drugalcdep.2011.07.007

[32] Elkashef AM, Rawson RA, Anderson AL, Li SH, Holmes T, Smith EV, et al. Bupropion for the treatment of methamphetamine dependence. Neuropsychopharmacology. 2008;**33**(5):1162-1170. DOI: 10.1038/sj.npp.1301481

[33] Kneebusch J, Farhadian S. Bupropion in comorbid post-traumatic stress disorder and methamphetamine use disorder. Journal of Pharmacy Practice. 2025;**38**(1):208-211. DOI: 10.1177/08971900241276698

[34] Srisurapanont M, Likhitsathian S, Suttajit S, Maneeton N, Maneeton B, Oon-Arom A, et al. Efficacy and dropout rates of antipsychotic medications for methamphetamine psychosis: A systematic review and network meta-analysis. Drug and Alcohol Dependence. 2021;**219**:108467. DOI: 10.1016/j.drugalcdep.2020.108467

[35] Boonlue T, Suwanmajo S, Suansanae T. PM293. Efficacy and safety of aripiprazole for maintenance treatment of methamphetamine dependence following methamphetamine psychosis: A naturalistic retrospective study. The International Journal of Neuropsychopharmacology. 2016;**19**(Suppl 1):4-5. DOI: 10.1093/ijnp/pyw041.293. eCollection 2016 Jun

[36] Chan B, Freeman M, Kondo K, Ayers C, Montgomery J, Paynter R, et al. Pharmacotherapy for methamphetamine/amphetamine use disorder—A systematic review and meta-analysis. Addiction. 2019;**114**(12):2122-2136. DOI: 10.1111/add.14755

[37] McKetin R, Dean OM, Turner A, Kelly PJ, Quinn B, Lubman DI, et al. N-acetylcysteine (NAC) for methamphetamine dependence: A randomised controlled trial. EClinicalMedicine. 2021;**38**:101005. DOI: 10.1016/j.eclinm.2021.101005

[38] Elkashef A, Kahn R, Yu E, Iturriaga E, Li SH, Anderson A, et al. Topiramate for the treatment of methamphetamine addiction: A multi-center placebo-controlled trial. Addiction. 2012;**107**(7):1297-1306. DOI: 10.1111/j.1360-0443.2011.03771.x

[39] Moghaddam Sadegh A, Nazarinasab M, Behrouzian F, Rostami H,

Mehrabi M. The effectiveness of topiramate in the treatment of amphetamine and methamphetamine use disorder: A randomized controlled trial. Iranian Journal of Psychiatry. 2023;**18**(4):371-379. DOI: 10.18502/ijps.v18i4.13624

[40] Hossain MK, Hassanza-deganroudsari M, Nurgali K, Apostolopoulos V. Vaccine development against methamphetamine drug addiction. Expert Review of Vaccines. 2020;**19**(12):1105-1114. DOI: 10.1080/14760584.2020.1857738

[41] Hossain MK, Davidson M, Feehan J, Deraos G, Nurgali K, Matsoukas J, et al. Development of methamphetamine conjugated vaccine through hapten design: In vitro and in vivo characterization. Vaccines (Basel). 2023;**11**(2). DOI: 10.3390/vaccines11020340

[42] da Silva MCM, de Souza Ferreira LP, Giustina AD. Could immunotherapy be a hope for addiction treatment? Clinics (São Paulo, Brazil). 2024;**79**:100347. DOI: 10.1016/j.clinsp.2024.100347

[43] Lee NK, Rawson RA. A systematic review of cognitive and behavioural therapies for methamphetamine dependence. Drug and Alcohol Review. 2008;**27**(3):309-317. DOI: 10.1080/09595230801919494

[44] AshaRani PV, Hombali A, Seow E, Ong WJ, Tan JH, Subramaniam M. Non-pharmacological interventions for methamphetamine use disorder: A systematic review. Drug and Alcohol Dependence. 2020;**212**:108060. DOI: 10.1016/j.drugalcdep.2020.108060

[45] Stuart AM, Baker AL, Denham AMJ, Lee NK, Hall A, Oldmeadow C, et al. Psychological treatment for methamphetamine use and associated psychiatric symptom outcomes: A systematic review. Journal of Substance Abuse Treatment. 2020;**109**:61-79. DOI: 10.1016/j.jsat.2019.09.005

[46] Elison-Davies S, Newsome J, Jones A, Davies G, Ward J. Associations between psychosocial risk factors, and changes in substance dependence and psychosocial functioning, during engagement with digital cognitive behavioral therapy for methamphetamine use: Use of 'Breaking Free from Substance Abuse' by incarcerated people during the COVID-19 pandemic. Health Justice. 2022;**10**(1):28. DOI: 10.1186/s40352-022-00190-w

[47] Chen T, Chen L, Li S, Du J, Su H, Jiang H, et al. Virtual digital psychotherapist app-based treatment in patients with methamphetamine use disorder (Echo-APP): Single-arm pilot feasibility and efficacy study. JMIR mHealth and uHealth. 2023;**11**:e40373. DOI: 10.2196/40373

[48] Brown HD, DeFulio A. Contingency management for the treatment of methamphetamine use disorder: A systematic review. Drug and Alcohol Dependence. 2020;**216**:108307. DOI: 10.1016/j.drugalcdep.2020.108307

[49] Chmiel J, Malinowska A, Rybakowski F, Leszek J. The effectiveness of mindfulness in the treatment of methamphetamine addiction symptoms: Does neuroplasticity play a role? Brain Sciences. 2024;**14**(4):1-28. DOI: 10.3390/brainsci14040320

[50] Rawson RA, Chudzynski J, Mooney L, Gonzales R, Ang A, Dickerson D, et al. Impact of an exercise intervention on methamphetamine use outcomes post-residential treatment care. Drug and Alcohol Dependence. 2015;**156**:21-28. DOI: 10.1016/j.drugalcdep.2015.08.029

[51] Xu C, Zhang Z, Hou D, Wang G, Li C, Ma X, et al. Effects of exercise interventions on negative emotions, cognitive performance and drug craving in methamphetamine addiction. Frontiers in Psychiatry. 2024;**15**:1402533. DOI: 10.3389/fpsyt.2024.1402533

[52] Aryan N, Banafshe HR, Farnia V, Shakeri J, Alikhani M, Rahimi H, et al. The therapeutic effects of methylphenidate and matrix-methylphenidate on addiction severity, craving, relapse and mental health in the methamphetamine use disorder. Substance Abuse Treatment, Prevention, and Policy. 2020;**15**(1):72. DOI: 10.1186/s13011-020-00317-y

[53] Kamp F, Proebstl L, Hager L, Schreiber A, Riebschläger M, Neumann S, et al. Effectiveness of methamphetamine abuse treatment: Predictors of treatment completion and comparison of two residential treatment programs. Drug and Alcohol Dependence. 2019;**201**:8-15. DOI: 10.1016/j.drugalcdep.2019.04.010

[54] Kamp F, Hager L, Proebstl L, Schreiber A, Riebschläger M, Neumann S, et al. 12- and 18-month follow-up after residential treatment of methamphetamine dependence: Influence of treatment drop-out and different treatment concepts. Journal of Psychiatric Research. 2020;**129**:103-110. DOI: 10.1016/j.jpsychires.2020.05.029

[55] Chang CH, Liou MF, Liu CY, Lu WH, Chen SJ. Efficacy of repetitive transcranial magnetic stimulation in patients with methamphetamine use disorder: A systematic review and meta-analysis of double-blind randomized controlled trials. Frontiers in Psychiatry. 2022;**13**:904252. DOI: 10.3389/fpsyt.2022.904252

[56] Rezvanian S, Saraei M, Mohajeri H, Hassani-Abharian P. The effect of different transcranial direct current stimulation (tDCS) protocols on drug craving and cognitive functions in methamphetamine addicts. Basic and Clinical Neuroscience. 2022;**13**(3):349-355. DOI: 10.32598/bcn.13.2.1929.1

[57] Fattahi M, Eskandari K, Riahi E, Khosrowabadi R, Haghparast A. Distinct suppressing effects of deep brain stimulation in the orbitofrontal cortex on the development, extinction, and reinstatement of methamphetamine-seeking behaviors. Life Sciences. 2023;**322**:121613. DOI: 10.1016/j.lfs.2023.121613

[58] Chen YH, Yang J, Wu H, Beier KT, Sawan M. Challenges and future trends in wearable closed-loop neuromodulation to efficiently treat methamphetamine addiction. Frontiers in Psychiatry. 2023;**14**:1085036. DOI: 10.3389/fpsyt.2023.1085036

[59] Tian W, Zhao D, Ding J, Zhan S, Zhang Y, Etkin A, et al. An electroencephalographic signature predicts craving for methamphetamine. Cell Reports Medicine. 2024;**5**(1):101347. DOI: 10.1016/j.xcrm.2023.101347

[60] Liu M, Si Z. An update: Epigenetic mechanisms underlying methamphetamine addiction. Frontiers in Cell and Development Biology. 2024;**12**:1494557. DOI: 10.3389/fcell.2024.1494557

Chapter 4

New Nicotine Delivery Devices and Their Role in Smoking Cessation and Tobacco Harm Reduction Strategies

Josep M. Ramon-Torrell

Abstract

Tobacco use is the leading risk factor for diseases with the highest incidence and mortality rates. Tobacco control policies addressing the main determinants of tobacco consumption, alongside traditional smoking cessation methods, have generally shown poor results, with relatively low cessation rates worldwide. For these reasons, it is crucial to adopt innovative strategies for smoking cessation while implementing changes in policies to reduce prevalence. The emergence of new nicotine delivery devices, which are less harmful than conventional tobacco, could potentially improve cessation rates and reduce the population-level impact of tobacco use. New nicotine delivery devices, such as electronic cigarettes, heated tobacco products, and nicotine pouches, offer innovative alternatives. A common feature among these devices is that none produce toxic components in amounts comparable to those found in conventional combustible tobacco smoke. Although the regulatory and safety aspects of these devices are still under debate by authorities worldwide, they have demonstrated effectiveness in population-level smoking cessation. Their role in reducing the harms of tobacco use is increasingly recognized in tobacco control policies. Integrating these new nicotine delivery devices into existing smoking cessation programs using standardized interventions may help address some challenges and explore new combinations that could prove more effective than current treatments.

Keywords: nicotine addiction, nicotine devices, smoking cessation, tobacco harm reduction, tobacco control

1. Introduction

Tobacco consumption is the leading cause of preventable deaths worldwide, significantly impacting public health across different countries. According to the World Health Organization (WHO), tobacco kills over eight million people annually, of which seven million are direct smokers, and the remainder are passive smokers [1].

The most significant impact of tobacco consumption is observed in the cardiovascular and respiratory systems. Smoking is a major risk factor for heart disease, strokes, and chronic obstructive pulmonary disease (COPD) [2]. Additionally, tobacco has been identified as the primary cause of lung cancer, responsible for approximately 85% of cases globally [3]. Other forms of cancer, such as those affecting the mouth, throat, esophagus, and pancreas, are also closely linked to smoking [4].

Tobacco has become the second most widely used psychoactive substance in the world, with nearly one billion smokers globally [5]. Despite a decline in its prevalence, particularly in Western countries, tobacco consumption has increased in low- and middle-income countries.

For much of the twentieth century, tobacco consumption was viewed as a behavior or habit chosen by the smoker, and the concept of "addiction" was not adopted. In the last quarter of that century, significant advancements were made in understanding the effects of tobacco on health and the role of nicotine as an addictive substance. People smoke for nicotine, which is responsible for the persistence of tobacco use and serves as the vehicle for inhaling all the harmful products present in tobacco smoke that cause various related diseases.

Why is tobacco recognized as an addictive substance? Could nicotine-addicted tobacco consumers reduce their risk of disease without giving up nicotine? Can we separate nicotine consumption from tobacco use? These are some of the key questions public health authorities around the world are addressing to prioritize reducing tobacco consumption, improving population health, and, fundamentally, decreasing the prevalence of smoking and protecting future generations [6].

The understanding of tobacco and nicotine's roles, alongside the concept of addiction, has completely changed the therapeutic approach to smokers, now considered nicotine-addicted patients. This shift facilitated the development of the first nicotine delivery products, which helped manage the physical symptoms of addiction and support tobacco cessation.

In recent years, various new nicotine delivery products have been developed. These products, on the one hand, help control nicotine withdrawal symptoms like traditional products, and on the other, reduce some of the harmful effects of cigarettes among smokers who are unable to quit entirely. New nicotine delivery devices, known as electronic nicotine delivery systems (ENDS), have emerged as an alternative to traditional nicotine replacement therapy (NRT) methods, such as nicotine gums and patches, with the less impactful SNUS.

In recent decades, the field of tobacco cessation has evolved beyond traditional products, with the introduction of non-nicotine options like bupropion and varenicline. Simultaneously, new nicotine delivery products without tobacco have emerged, including electronic cigarettes and pouches that allow nicotine release without combustion, along with heated (not burned) tobacco products (HTPs).

Interest in ENDS has grown due to their potential to assist in smoking cessation and reduce the harm associated with tobacco use among smokers who cannot completely quit. Although not without controversy—due to concerns about their long-term safety and appeal to young non-smokers—ENDS represent an important tool in modern tobacco control strategies. Understanding their mechanism of action is essential, as it involves the role of nicotine in tobacco addiction and its effects on the human body.

This chapter will explore the different types of devices available, their mechanisms of action, and their effectiveness in the context of tobacco cessation and harm reduction, evaluating both their benefits and limitations.

DOI: http://dx.doi.org/10.5772/intechopen.1009109

Although the chapter does not aim to provide a systematic review, the literature has been reviewed regarding the existence of associations between nicotine use and the risk of various diseases. Additionally, the effects of NGPs (nicotine delivery products) on users' health, their mechanisms of action, and existing evidence on their role in smoking cessation and harm reduction strategies have been examined. The search strategy was based on locating relevant articles on the topic using Google Scholar and PubMed databases. The keywords used in the search were: "nicotine," "electronic nicotine delivery systems," "nicotine effects", "harm reduction," and "nicotine addiction." The studies located were prioritized based on their impact and publication in peer-reviewed journals in English.

2. Nicotine

Nicotine is the main psychoactive component in tobacco smoke. Russell, the pioneer of nicotine replacement therapy, stated that "people smoke for the nicotine and have difficulty quitting tobacco use because they become addicted to it and die due to the toxic components present in tobacco smoke after combustion" [7].

Nicotine is a tertiary amine composed of a pyridine and a pyrrolidine ring, (S)-nicotine, found primarily in tobacco leaves. It belongs to the alkaloid group, which contains nitrogen, granting it the ability to interact with specific receptors in the human nervous system. This interaction is crucial for understanding its addictive potential and pharmacological effects [8]. When smoking, nicotine is rapidly absorbed through the oral mucosa and respiratory tract, reaching the central nervous system within 10–15 seconds after inhalation. This rapid onset contributes significantly to its high addictive potential [6].

Nicotine quickly binds to nicotinic acetylcholine receptors (nAChRs) in the brain, mimicking the action of acetylcholine, as will be detailed in subsequent sections. These receptors are associated with multiple central nervous system functions, including the regulation of attention, learning, memory, and mood [9]. Their activation triggers the release of dopamine, a neurotransmitter involved in the reward system. This largely explains nicotine's addictive potential, as dopamine induces sensations of pleasure and positive reinforcement.

The interaction of nicotine with these neurochemical systems is complex, and chronic consumption can lead to receptor desensitization, causing the need for higher doses to achieve the same effects, this process results in tolerance and dependence [10].

2.1 Neurobiology of nicotine addiction

Nicotine addiction is a complex process involving both neurobiological mechanisms and psychological factors. Multiple lines of research [8, 11, 12] have demonstrated that nicotine reinforcement is primarily controlled by two pathways associated with reward or aversion. The rewarding properties of nicotine involve the mesolimbic system, where dopamine is released from the ventral tegmental area (VTA) to the nucleus accumbens. Conversely, nicotine's aversive properties, which regulate withdrawal symptoms, are linked to the projection of the habenula's medial fasciculus retroflexus to the interpeduncular nucleus. However, other brain regions, such as the prefrontal cortex, ventral pallidum (VP), nucleus tractus solitarius, and insula, are also involved in various aspects of nicotine dependence. These brain areas are directly or indirectly interconnected as integrative circuits driving consumption-seeking behavior.

From a neurobiological perspective, nicotine addiction is mediated by the activation of nicotinic acetylcholine receptors (nAChRs). These receptors are widely distributed across different brain areas, including those involved in reward control, learning, and memory, such as the nucleus accumbens and VTA. When nicotine binds to these receptors, it triggers dopamine release in the nucleus accumbens, generating sensations of pleasure and positive reinforcement, thereby facilitating dependence [8]. Nicotine acts as an agonist at the nAChRs.

Neuronal nAChRs are composed of alpha (α) and beta (β) subunits arranged around a central pore, with subunits from α2 to α6 and β2 to β4, forming various combinations. Functionally, nAChR complexes can exist in three states—closed, open, and desensitized—which are dynamically regulated by exposure to their agonist. These functional states depend on the subunit sequence, the agonist's dose, and binding kinetics. When nicotine reaches the brain, binding to these receptors occurs within minutes, with the α4-β2 receptors showing the highest affinity for nicotine. This binding can last for hours [13–15].

The nAChRs are transmembrane proteins of the family of ionotropic receptors, and their activation depends on binding to a ligand, such as acetylcholine or nicotine. Once nicotine binds, the receptor opens an ion channel, allowing the influx of cations, primarily sodium and calcium, which depolarize the neuronal membrane and trigger an intracellular signaling cascade [16]. The activation of these receptors in the VTA is critical for addiction development, as they modulate the activity of dopaminergic neurons by stimulating dopamine release in the nucleus accumbens, a key region in the reward system; they play a central role in reinforcing nicotine use [17].

Dopamine is not the only neurotransmitter involved in nicotine addiction. The activation of nAChRs also induces the release of other neurotransmitters, such as glutamate, serotonin, and norepinephrine, which significantly influence behavior, including mood, alertness, and attention [18]. Glutamate is particularly important because it enhances the activity of dopaminergic neurons by amplifying dopamine release in response to nicotine, intensifying its addictive effect [10].

With chronic nicotine use, nAChRs experience desensitization, where they remain inactive despite continued nicotine presence, reducing their responsiveness. To compensate, the number of brain receptors increases (upregulation), contributing to tolerance and the need for higher doses to achieve the same effects [19]. Additionally, some components of tobacco smoke other than nicotine, such as monoamine oxidase, contribute to addiction by catalyzing the metabolism of dopamine, norepinephrine, and serotonin, effectively reducing nicotine metabolism [8].

2.2 The mesolimbic pathway of addiction

The mesolimbic circuit is a fundamental reinforcement system for behavior. Dopaminergic centers in the midbrain play a key role in arousal, motivation, cognition, motor function, and processes associated with reinforcement behaviors leading to reward. One of the dopaminergic pathways originates in the ventral tegmental area (VTA) of the midbrain and projects to the prefrontal cortex, as well as areas such as the olfactory tubercle, amygdala, septal region, striatum, and, most notably, the nucleus accumbens. The binding of nicotine to nAChRs in the VTA induces depolarization of dopaminergic neurons, increasing their activity and consequently the release of dopamine in the nucleus accumbens [20]. This structure plays a central role in the reward system, acting as a "switch" that generates feelings of pleasure and reinforcement upon dopamine release.

Continuous exposure to nicotine induces long-term changes in the brain, a process known as neuroadaptation, in which the brain adjusts to prolonged exposure. This phenomenon involves neurobiological modifications affecting the function of neurotransmitters, receptors, and brain circuits. Neuroadaptation underlies the development of tolerance, dependence, and withdrawal symptoms characteristic of addiction. These effects are particularly pronounced in neural systems involved in the reward system, especially the mesolimbic dopamine pathway, as well as other neurotransmitter systems such as glutamate, GABA, and acetylcholine [21]. Prolonged exposure also reduces the dopaminergic system's ability to release dopamine in the absence of the drug [22]. This process, called dopaminergic hypofunction, contributes to feelings of dysphoria and anhedonia during withdrawal periods, driving individuals to consume more nicotine to restore normal dopamine levels.

When nicotine use is interrupted, the lack of nAChR receptor stimulation and the dysfunction of the dopaminergic system result in withdrawal symptoms, including irritability, anxiety, difficulty concentrating, and anhedonia. These symptoms reflect the brain's inability to maintain normal neurochemical balance without nicotine [20].

Finally, it is important to emphasize the psychological component of tobacco addiction, which extends beyond nicotine itself and is influenced by environmental and social factors. Exposure to situations or stimuli associated with smoking can trigger intense cravings, even long after cessation [23].

In conclusion, nicotine addiction results from a complex interaction between neurobiological mechanisms, involving changes in the brain's reward systems and desensitization of nicotinic receptors, and psychological factors, such as positive and negative reinforcements and environmental influences. Understanding this interaction is essential for developing effective interventions to treat tobacco dependence.

3. Health risks associated with nicotine and NGPs

The most debated issues regarding new nicotine delivery devices (NGPs) are, first, the safety of these products and, second, their potential role as a gateway to conventional cigarettes among younger populations. Additionally, nicotine's addictive properties are often cited as a primary challenge to their use, which seems somewhat inconsistent given the substantial health impact of tobacco consumption on populations. It is indisputable that nicotine alone is not harmless, and its effects on various organs and systems are summarized in **Table 1**.

The key to the future fight against tobacco addiction lies in dissociating tobacco use from nicotine consumption, acknowledging the much lower health risks of nicotine compared to conventional cigarettes. Some experts (K. Fargeström, personal communication) suggest that while it is possible to eradicate or drastically reduce tobacco use in society, eliminating nicotine use altogether may be unlikely due to its psycho-stimulant effects.

One of the best population-level examples is the impact of SNUS use in Sweden. Sweden represents a unique and notable case in tobacco control, achieving a dramatic reduction in cigarette consumption through SNUS use and, consequently, a significant decline in tobacco-related disease prevalence [24]. Although not risk-free, SNUS has proven to be less harmful than conventional tobacco, particularly regarding

System	Immediate effects	Medium-term effects
Central nervous system	• Release of dopamine in the nucleus accumbens (feeling of pleasure) • Increased activation of nicotinic acetylcholine receptors (nAChR) • Increased alertness and concentration	• Desensitization of nAChR receptors • Increased tolerance and dependence • Changes in synaptic plasticity that facilitate addiction
Cardiovascular system	• Increased heart rate and blood pressure • Peripheral vasoconstriction (decreased blood flow to extremities)	• Persistent high blood pressure • Increased risk of arrhythmias and heart disease • Possible hardening of the arteries (arteriosclerosis)
Respiratory system	• Irritation of the airways • Increased breathing rate	• Decreased lung function • Increased inflammation in the airways • Increased risk of respiratory infections
Digestive system	• Reduced appetite • Stimulation of gastric acid secretion (possible stomach upset)	• Problems with digestion and absorption of nutrients • Increased risk of gastritis and gastric ulcers
Endocrine and metabolism	• Increased release of catecholamines (adrenaline and noradrenaline) • Increased basal metabolism	• Impaired glucose and insulin regulation • Possible development of insulin resistance • Weight loss in some chronic users
Skin and connective tissue	• Cutaneous vasoconstriction (temporarily paler skin)	• Decreased skin elasticity • Premature aging and possible chronic skin dehydration
Immune system	• Temporary suppression of some immune functions	• Impaired immune response • Increased susceptibility to infections and inflammatory diseases
Psychological effects	• Feeling of well-being or euphoria • Reduction of momentary anxiety	• Increased anxiety and stress in the absence of nicotine • Psychological dependence and withdrawal syndrome • Possible cognitive impairment in prolonged use

Table 1.
Immediate and medium-term effects of nicotine on the human body by specific body systems and mechanisms.

cardiovascular diseases and cancer. Swedish statistics support the hypothesis that transitioning from smoked tobacco to non-combustible tobacco—or nicotine use—could serve as a viable alternative to reduce tobacco's public health impact.

According to World Health Organization (WHO) reports, Sweden is the only country in the European Union where conventional tobacco use has fallen below 10% among adults, a rate remarkably lower than other European nations [25]. This shift is reflected in reduced rates of tobacco-related diseases and a decline in mortality attributed to these illnesses, with Sweden maintaining some of the lowest cancer and cardiovascular disease mortality rates in Europe, largely due to cigarette substitution with SNUS [26].

Separating the effects of nicotine from those of other components in tobacco smoke regarding disease risk is complex. This difficulty arises from the challenge of identifying study populations that use nicotine without a prior smoking history. Tobacco smoke contains over 7000 compounds, including toxic gases like carbon monoxide and ammonia, as well as carcinogens such as polycyclic aromatic hydrocarbons and tobacco-specific nitrosamines [27]. These compounds, along with nicotine, can interact and affect multiple organs and systems both immediately and over the medium and long term (**Table 1**).

A recent comprehensive review by Scherer et al. [28] evaluated the scientific evidence on the short- and long-term association of NGPs with specific diseases, drawing on both population studies and animal experiments. The synergy between nicotine and other components of tobacco smoke complicates efforts to identify nicotine's specific disease risks. The coexistence of combustion byproducts in tobacco can amplify nicotine's effects, particularly on the cardiovascular system. Some studies [27] have linked certain particles, such as aldehydes, to increased nicotine bioavailability, further complicating the assessment of nicotine's individual effects.

As noted, associating nicotine alone with disease risk is extremely challenging. Concerns about this association have grown in recent years with the emergence and impact of NGPs and other products that primarily contain nicotine.

3.1 Nicotine, NGPs, and cardiovascular risk

The specific role of nicotine in cardiovascular risk is a widely debated topic, primarily because nicotine is not the only biologically active component in the aerosols generated by e-cigarettes (ECs) and heated tobacco products (HTPs). Some studies [29] have proposed potential mechanisms linking nicotine and NGPs to cardiovascular risk, including endothelial dysfunction, vascular reactivity, and increased thrombogenesis (**Table 2**). These potential direct effects of nicotine must also be considered alongside those caused by other aerosol components, such as acrolein and other aldehydes. The aerosols from these devices contain ultrafine particles that are biologically active and can trigger inflammatory processes potentially associated with cardiovascular diseases (CVD).

A study conducted by Benowitz and Gourlay [30] evaluated the safety profile of traditional nicotine replacement therapy (NRT) products and concluded that the cardiovascular risk was small among users of these products. Moreover, they found no increased risk when used by patients with a history of CVD. Overall, these products were shown to provide substantial benefits by helping patients quit smoking.

Animal studies allow researchers to isolate nicotine's impact from other tobacco components and assess its effects on specific body systems. Experimental studies in animals, particularly rodents, have demonstrated that nicotine affects the cardiovascular system, including increasing blood pressure and heart rate. One study found that prolonged exposure to nicotine was associated with endothelial damage, myocardial hypertrophy, and changes in arterial elasticity [31]. Experimental evidence also shows that nicotine promotes oxidative stress in the cardiovascular system, contributing to the development of atherosclerosis and other vascular effects [31].

Effects	Conventional cigarette	NGPs
Oxidative stress	Induces	Induces lower level
Inflammation	Activate and promotes	Lower level
Cytotoxic effect	Cytotoxic effect	Effect may be milder
Thrombus formation	Support formation	Could support formation
Adapted from Klein et al. [29].		

Table 2.
Major effects of conventional cigarettes in comparison to next-generation nicotine products on the vascular wall.

This section on the nicotine-CVD association can be summarized using conclusions from two significant scientific reports [32, 33]:

- There is no evidence of an association between nicotine and coronary heart disease (CHD) or CVD.
- Strong evidence indicates that nicotine and NGPs increase heart rate.
- Limited evidence suggests that nicotine and ECs alter biomarkers of oxidative stress and increase endothelial dysfunction.
- There is no evidence that nicotine and ECs are associated with long-term changes in heart rate, blood pressure, or cardiac function.

3.2 Nicotine, NGPs, and cancer risk

The increasing use of novel nicotine delivery products (NGPs) has sparked a significant debate regarding their potential association with various types of cancer. Although the levels of carcinogens present in these products are significantly lower than in conventional cigarettes, traces of carcinogens have been identified in users of these devices [34].

The case of Sweden and SNUS offers a notable example: its use has not been associated with higher rates of lung, oral, or other cancers. In fact, Sweden has one of the lowest rates of lung cancer in Europe [24]. However, it is essential to note that SNUS is not an inhaled product and does not contain nitrosamines, meaning its results may not be directly extrapolable to NGPs, which generate aerosols. Even with low-dose exposure to carcinogens, the risks associated with aerosolized products need further investigation.

Experimental evidence shows that NGPs contain significantly lower amounts of carcinogenic compounds than conventional tobacco, potentially reducing cancer risks considerably. Nevertheless, there could still be associations with certain cancers, primarily respiratory and digestive [35]. Currently, there are very few studies examining the potential cancer risk of NGPs in humans, and no substantial evidence suggests that these products significantly increase cancer risk. This aligns with the view that nicotine itself is not a primary driver of carcinogenesis [28].

Although nicotine is not directly carcinogenic, some animal studies have demonstrated that it can act as a tumor promoter by facilitating cell proliferation and angiogenesis, particularly when combined with other carcinogens. For instance, when nicotine was administered alongside polycyclic aromatic hydrocarbons (PAHs) in animal models, a significant increase in the growth and progression of lung and pancreatic tumors was observed [36].

Heated tobacco products (HTPs), which warm tobacco without full combustion, reduce the release of certain carcinogens in their aerosols. However, preliminary studies suggest that these aerosols still contain toxic compounds, such as PAHs and tobacco-specific nitrosamines (TSNAs), albeit at lower levels than conventional cigarettes. These compounds may still pose a cancer risk [37]. **Table 3** provides an overview of the concentrations of various components in conventional tobacco smoke versus NGP aerosols.

From an experimental standpoint, nicotine has demonstrated pro-carcinogenic potential primarily through its interaction with nicotinic acetylcholine receptors (nAChRs) present in various cell types. Activation of these receptors can promote cell proliferation, inhibit apoptosis, and stimulate angiogenesis—factors that collectively contribute to tumor development and progression [38].

3.3 Nicotine, NGPs, and risk of non-cancer pulmonary diseases

It is estimated that 35–45% of patients with chronic obstructive pulmonary disease (COPD) are current smokers, while only 20% have never smoked. Among asthma patients, the prevalence of smoking is similar to that of the general population [39, 40]. Evidence strongly supports that smoking cessation strategies for COPD patients improve prognosis and significantly slow the deterioration of lung function.

Chemical	Conventional cigarette (smoke)	Electronic cigarette (aerosol)	Heated tobacco (aerosol)
Nicotine	1–3 mg/cigarette	0.5–20 mg/mL in e-liquids	1–2 mg/use
Tar	10–15 mg/cigarette	Absent	Absent
Carbon monoxide (CO)	20–30 mg/cigarette	Absent	0.5–2 mg/use
Formaldehyde	20–100 μg/cigarette	0.1–5 μg/inhalation	5–15 μg/use
Acrolein	10–140 μg/cigarette	0.7–8 μg/inhalation	8–20 μg/use
Acetaldehyde	1000–1500 μg/cigarette	20–50 μg/inhalation	60–120 μg/use
Tobacco-specific nitrosamines (TSNAs)	100–250 ng/cigarette	1–30 μg/inhalation	10–30 ng/use
Polycyclic aromatic hydrocarbons (PAHs)	100–200 ng/cigarette	Absent	Absent
Heavy metals (lead, cadmium, nickel)	0.1–0.2 μg/cigarette	0.001–0.02 μg/ inhalation	0.05–0.1 μg/use
Volatile organic compounds	1000–2000 μg/cigarette	20–200 μg/inhalation	100–300 μg/use
Benzene	200–400 μg/cigarette	<1 μg/inhalation	1–5 μg/use
Glycerol and propylene glycol	Absent	100–400 mg/ inhalation	50–150 mg/use

Table 3.
Typical concentrations and approximate ranges of some substances present in cigarette smoke.

The role of new nicotine delivery products (NGPs) in relation to their aerosol generation for patients at risk of COPD or those already diagnosed has sparked considerable controversy. Certain evidence suggests that repeated exposure to these aerosols may be associated with chronic lung inflammation, mucus hypersecretion, increased pulmonary resistance, and tissue damage, all of which are linked to COPD progression [41]. Vaping and the use of other inhaled NGPs could potentially induce respiratory diseases through mechanisms similar to those observed in conventional tobacco smokers [42, 43]. In contrast, oral NGPs, such as SNUS or nicotine pouches, do not have direct effects on the respiratory tract.

A recent review by Morjaria et al. [44] analyzed 16 observational studies investigating potential associations between electronic cigarette (EC) use and COPD. The review did not identify any studies examining the role of heated tobacco products (HTPs). Most of the reviewed articles were cross-sectional and reported significant associations between EC use and COPD-like symptoms. However, as noted by the authors, most EC users studied were either former smokers currently using ECs or dual users (conventional tobacco smokers and EC users). This limits the ability to establish true associations from a cross-sectional perspective.

The major strategy for improving prognosis in COPD patients is smoking cessation. However, many patients struggle to quit, showing high relapse rates, and continue smoking despite their symptoms. The use of NGPs to maintain abstinence could be a viable option for these patients, as they reduce the risks associated with conventional tobacco.

4. New nicotine delivery devices

In recent years, new nicotine delivery devices have emerged as alternatives to conventional tobacco use, significantly transforming the market and offering potential support for smoking cessation. These devices hold promise in the fight against tobacco-related harm, although their role in tobacco control policies remains highly debated. On one side, proponents argue that these devices should be considered a potential tool for harm reduction, as they offer significantly reduced exposure to the toxic substances generated by combustible tobacco. On the other hand, critics claim that they foster nicotine dependency, act as a gateway to conventional tobacco use, and risk leading non-smokers to nicotine addiction.

These nicotine-generating products (NGPs) are designed to deliver nicotine without combustion—or at much lower temperatures than conventional tobacco—thus eliminating the primary source of harmful toxins responsible for the diseases associated with traditional smoking. By removing combustion, exposure to these harmful substances is significantly reduced, though not entirely eliminated.

Although these products are notably less toxic compared to conventional cigarettes, long-term safety studies remain insufficient, despite increasingly promising evidence. Preliminary research suggests that certain components of the aerosols produced—such as glycerol and propylene glycol in electronic cigarettes (ECs)—may induce lung inflammation after prolonged exposure. However, the absolute risk posed by these new products is much lower than that of traditional tobacco products [45].

From a regulatory perspective, approaches to these products vary widely by country. Some nations have incorporated NGPs into harm-reduction policies, while others have imposed stricter regulations, refusing to promote them as safer alternatives. These stricter policies cite concerns about nicotine addiction, youth use, and the lack of definitive evidence regarding their long-term impact on tobacco control efforts [46].

Despite these ongoing controversies, as previously highlighted, it is clear that these products have significant potential to reduce the harm caused by tobacco use—provided they are used appropriately and regulated effectively. This includes careful oversight of their use among youth and specific products, particularly ECs and heated tobacco products [47].

4.1 Types of ENDS

These products include electronic cigarettes, heated tobacco devices, and oral nicotine products such as nicotine pouches. While their designs vary, they all share the goal of delivering nicotine in a more controlled manner, minimizing exposure to the toxic compounds found in tobacco smoke.

4.1.1 Electronic cigarettes

Electronic cigarettes (ECs) were the first widely available alternatives to combustible tobacco—excluding SNUS. Hon Lik, a Chinese pharmacist, created the first modern EC, which was initially marketed in China in 2003 and introduced in the U.S. and Europe in 2007 (**Table 4**). The term "EC" refers to a device containing a central mechanism that vaporizes a liquid (e-liquid), typically composed of propylene glycol, vegetable glycerol, nicotine, and flavorings. These devices do not contain tobacco or involve its combustion.

Since their inception, ECs have evolved considerably, and they are now classified into four generations:

- First generation: These devices resembled cigarettes in size and shape and were available in disposable or rechargeable formats (**Figure 1**). The original ECs featured a three-piece design comprising an atomizer, battery, and fluid tank.

- Second generation (Tank systems): These ECs introduced refillable tanks and larger batteries, enabling greater customization in terms of power and vapor production. They included a button that must be pressed continuously during inhalation and were also rechargeable (**Figure 1**).

- Third generation (Mods): Mods departed from the cigarette-like appearance, incorporating more powerful batteries and advanced configurations. These devices allowed users to adjust temperature and voltage to optimize their experience.

- Fourth generation (Pod systems): The most recent development, pod systems, use pre-filled e-liquid capsules (pods). They are compact, easy to use, and highly popular. These devices often include automatic temperature controls and support advanced configurations, such as sub-ohm purifiers with adjustable airflow. The use of microporous ceramics for wicking enhances heating efficiency, though its impact on chemical emissions is not fully understood [48]. The liquids used in pod systems typically contain high nicotine concentrations (~50–60 mg/mL) and an acid that protonates nicotine, reducing the harshness of the aerosol [49].

Product	Description	Delivery method	Year of marketing	Advantages and disadvantages
Electronic Cigarette (e-cig)	An electronic device that heats a liquid (e-liquid) with nicotine to generate an aerosol.	E-liquid vaporization	~2003 (China); 2007 (EE. U.S.)	Advantages: Lower production of toxic substances compared to tobacco. Disadvantages: Possibility of generating formaldehyde, dependence on batteries.
Heated Tobacco System (HTP)	It heats tobacco at a lower temperature without combustion, generating an aerosol with nicotine and tobacco flavor.	Solid Tobacco Heating	~2014 (Japan and others)	Advantages: Reduced exposure to combustion products. Cons: It still produces some toxic substances, and its long-term safety is under evaluation.
SNUS	Pasteurized powdered tobacco placed under the upper lip, common in Sweden.	Sublingual absorption	~1980s (modern in Sweden)	Advantages: Reduced risk compared to smoking. Cons: Can cause gum and tooth injuries, and nicotine dependence.
Nicotine Pouch	Small, tobacco-free pouches with synthetic nicotine that you place in your mouth under your lip.	Oral absorption	~2016	Advantages: No tobacco, lower oral risks compared to snus. Cons: Potential for abuse, lack of long-term studies.

Table 4.
Classification of new nicotine delivery products according to their characteristics.

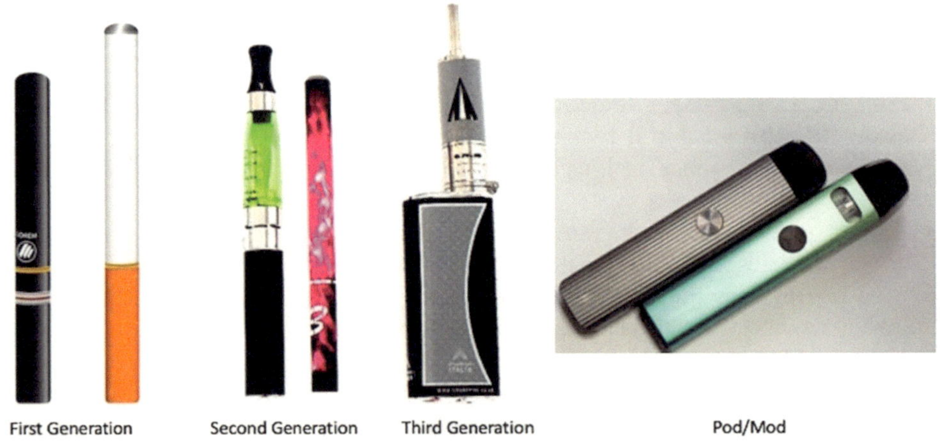

Figure 1.
Different types of electronic cigarettes.

4.1.2 Heated tobacco products

Heated tobacco products (HTPs) are a newer category of tobacco devices with limited toxicological data. HTPs heat reconstituted tobacco to approximately 350°C to produce a nicotine-containing aerosol. This is in contrast to traditional combustible cigarettes (TCCs), which reach temperatures of up to 900°C during burning.

HTPs were developed as a harm-reduction strategy compared to conventional cigarettes. The primary difference between HTPs and conventional cigarettes is the heating process versus combustion. Tobacco companies claim that due to this difference, HTP aerosols contain fewer toxic chemicals than conventional cigarette smoke [50].

HTPs are classified into two categories based on their technology:

1. Internal heating devices: These use an electric heater to heat processed tobacco units (sticks) to temperatures between 250°C and 350°C, enough to generate an aerosol without combustion (e.g., IQOS and Ploom).

2. External heating devices: These heat the tobacco using an external source, such as an induction system.

The principle behind HTPs is to avoid the combustion of tobacco, which occurs at temperatures above 600°C in conventional cigarettes. In HTPs, tobacco is heated just enough to produce an aerosol containing nicotine and other compounds, delivering a sensory experience similar to smoking [51]. While the nicotine release varies by device, concentrations are generally similar to or slightly lower than those of conventional cigarettes.

HTPs generate significantly lower levels of toxic compounds compared to traditional cigarettes. However, as noted earlier, they do not entirely eliminate exposure to these substances [52].

4.1.3 Nicotine pouches

Recently (**Table 4**), a new class of non-combustible nicotine products, known as oral nicotine pouches (ONPs), has emerged. ONPs are pre-portioned pouches resembling traditional snus, developed as a safer alternative to traditional tobacco and snus. Their introduction is linked to the growing interest in harm reduction associated with tobacco use and providing options for smokers who cannot or do not wish to give up nicotine. The first nicotine pouches were marketed in Sweden and other Scandinavian countries where snus usage was already established. Since their global market introduction post-2016, their classification and regulation have varied significantly across countries.

Some countries classify ONPs as nicotine replacement therapies and regulate them as medicinal products (e.g., Finland, Spain, and Australia), while others classify them as tobacco products (e.g., Brazil and the United States). In some countries, ONP sales are banned or proposed to be banned (e.g., the Netherlands, Belgium, and Singapore) or remain unregulated (e.g., Germany, Sweden, and the United Kingdom).

ONPs are small pouches similar to traditional snus but do not contain tobacco. They are composed of a blend of synthetic nicotine, plant fibers, humectants, and flavorings. The main types differ based on their nicotine content:

- *Low concentration*: 2–4 mg of nicotine per pouch.

- *Moderate concentration*: 6–8 mg.

- *High concentration*: 10–15 mg or more.

This variety allows users to adapt the product to their needs. They are available in different formats, including slim (more discreet and comfortable) and regular (standard size, similar to snus). Both formats are offered in various flavors.

Their use is simple and similar to snus: the pouch is placed between the upper lip and the gum, releasing nicotine through the oral mucosa into the bloodstream. Absorption is slower compared to inhaled methods.

5. NGPs for smoking cessation

Helping smokers quit tobacco use is one of the main challenges in tobacco control policies, as success rates with traditional methods like nicotine replacement therapy (NRT) or non-nicotine drugs remain low. NGPs, such as ECs, HTPs, and nicotine pouches, have emerged as alternatives to conventional cigarettes and are being evaluated as substitutes for traditional cessation methods. However, their effectiveness compared to traditional methods remains a topic of debate.

Of all NGPs, ECs are the most studied from a clinical perspective, with strong evidence supporting their role in increasing quit rates (**Table 5**). Meta-analyses by Hartmann-Boyce et al. [53] and Lindson et al. [55] demonstrated higher efficacy of nicotine-containing ECs compared to placebo and NRT (RR 1.59, 95% CI 1.29–1.93). Comparisons with varenicline showed moderate evidence favoring varenicline (**Table 5**). A randomized controlled trial (RCT) in the United Kingdom reported 1-year abstinence rates of 18% among EC users, compared to 9.9% for those using traditional NRTs [56]. Moderate-certainty evidence, limited by imprecision, suggests that nicotine ECs increase quit rates compared to non-nicotine ECs (RR 1.46, 95% CI 1.09–1.96) [53]. However, ECs present specific challenges, including variability in nicotine delivery between models and the potential for dual use.

HTPs have limited evidence supporting their use as a smoking cessation aid. Most available comparisons are industry-sponsored studies, which report a 14% quit rate at six months among smokers using HTPs versus a 5% quit rate among those with no assistance [57]. A meta-analysis by Tattan-Birch et al. [58], which reviewed 13 studies with an average smoker follow-up of 13 weeks, found no differences in adverse effects between HTPs and conventional cigarettes. Caponnetto et al. [59], in a randomized study comparing ECs and HTPs, reported continuous abstinence rates between weeks 4 and 12 of 39.1% for EC users and 30.8% for HTP users, with no significant differences between the two products.

Product	RR efficacy vs. placebo	RR vs. NRT	RR vs. Vareniclina	Studies or meta-analyses
E-Cigarettes	1.7–2.5	1.3–1.9	0.7–0.9	Hartmann-Boyce et al. [53]
Heated Tobacco	1.5–2.4	Limited Comparison	N/A	Hartmann-Boyce et al. [53]
Pouches de Nicotine	1.5–2.3	N/A	N/A	Lunell et al. [54]

Table 5.
Efficacy of the different new nicotine delivery devices for smoking cessation.

Although nicotine pouches are relatively new to the market, some evidence supports their efficacy for smoking cessation. In a clinical trial by Lunell et al. [54], nicotine pouches demonstrated higher quit rates compared to placebo (**Table 5**), particularly among smokers with low to moderate nicotine dependence. However, no studies have directly compared pouches to other cessation methods. Observational studies conducted in Nordic countries, where these products have a high penetration as a substitute for snus, suggest they may play an important role in smoking cessation.

6. NPGs and harm reduction

Harm reduction and harm minimization are widely used approaches in public health to address risk behaviors. These terms are often used interchangeably but define distinct concepts with different practical implications. Both strategies aim to reduce the impact of certain behaviors without necessarily eliminating them. In the context of tobacco, they recognize that total abstinence may not always be the goal. Historically, efforts to control and address smoking have focused on strategies like total cessation, preventing initiation, and implementing regulatory and restrictive policies. However, these two newer approaches have gained interest in recent years.

Harm reduction focuses on decreasing the consequences associated with tobacco use, even if complete cessation is not achieved (**Table 6**). This approach assumes that not all smokers can or want to quit but may benefit from less harmful alternatives, such as NPGs. In this case, harm reduction involves providing nicotine outside of tobacco use, avoiding nicotine abstinence while eliminating the primary source of toxic substances: tobacco smoke.

Harm minimization, on the other hand, has a broader goal (**Table 6**), encompassing not only the reduction of the negative impact of smoking but also a decrease in the prevalence of tobacco use. This strategy includes prevention, regulation, cessation promotion, and addressing the social and economic environments in which tobacco consumption occurs. Minimization seeks to protect not only smokers but also non-smokers by reducing their exposure to tobacco smoke.

New nicotine delivery products (NPLNs), such as electronic cigarettes, heated tobacco products (HTPs), and nicotine pouches, are potential alternatives for inclusion in harm reduction policies. However, unlike their use as smoking cessation aids,

Aspect	Harm reduction	Harm minimization
Main objective	Reduce the negative consequences of consumption.	Reduce both the prevalence of consumption and its consequences.
Focus on abstinence	It is not a priority; continued use of nicotine products is permitted.	It can include abstinence as the end goal.
Level of intervention	Focused on the individual and their choices.	It includes measures at the social, environmental, and structural levels.
Products and strategies	E-cigarettes, heated tobacco.	Smoking bans, anti-smoking campaigns.
Short-term impact	Reduced immediate risk of disease.	Long-term prevalence reduction.

Table 6.
Comparison of harm reduction strategies in smoking.

their long-term efficacy as alternatives to conventional cigarettes, along with their associated risks, remains a subject of debate. The Swedish example with snus, given its similarities as a non-inhaled nicotine delivery method, could support the use of nicotine pouches as a harm reduction alternative.

6.1 Evidence supporting harm reduction

Some studies provide evidence of the potential role of nicotine delivery devices in harm reduction. A report by the Royal College of Physicians suggests that the use of electronic cigarettes poses less than 5% of the risk associated with conventional cigarette use [60]. A cross-sectional study examining biomarkers of exposure among 181 participants in various groups found that exclusive EC users had significantly lower levels of toxic compounds compared to other groups (conventional tobacco, HTPs, dual use, and NRT), equivalent to a 95% reduction in toxicants compared to conventional cigarettes [61]. Moderate evidence also suggests lower levels of harmful compounds in HTP users compared to conventional cigarette smokers [58].

6.2 Questions regarding the implementation of NPGs in harm reduction

The incorporation of NPGs into harm reduction strategies raises several long-term impact questions:

1. *Impact on smoking prevalence*: Evidence from countries like Japan and Sweden suggests that NPGs can partially displace conventional cigarette use. However, their impact would also depend on the regulatory and promotional policies implemented.

2. *Risks associated with dual use*: Many smokers use these new products alongside conventional cigarettes, which could diminish the potential benefits. Nonetheless, partial replacement of smoking with NPGs may reduce toxicant exposure, although no studies have conclusively supported this claim.

3. *Adoption by vulnerable populations*: The adoption of NPGs by smokers, especially in low-income populations, could significantly reduce smoking-related diseases.

4. *Long-term risk monitoring*: Long-term studies are required to evaluate the impact of NPGs on harm reduction strategies.

7. Gateway hypothesis

The use of electronic devices, such as electronic cigarettes and heated tobacco products, has increased in recent years among younger populations, raising concerns in tobacco control policies that these devices might become a gateway to cigarette consumption for those who have never smoked conventional tobacco.

As we have discussed in the previous sections, these new devices offer clear advantages in reducing the harm caused by conventional tobacco among smokers. However, we should also consider the potential downsides—primarily of inhaled devices—particularly their role among young people. According to data from the National Institute on Drug Abuse (NIDA) in the U.S. [62], electronic cigarettes have become the primary form of nicotine consumption among young people. This is due to factors such as advertising, flavors, ease of access, and the (accurate) perception of a lower health risk compared to conventional cigarettes.

The main argument put forth by proponents of the gateway hypothesis is that the use of these devices might be adopted by individuals who have never smoked before, that is, by those who have never used nicotine. This concern is based on the idea that their use among young people could serve as a gateway to cigarette smoking, much like marijuana was once claimed to act as a gateway to more harmful drugs—an argument that has since been discredited [63, 64]. These hypotheses rest on the association between young people using these devices and their subsequent use of conventional cigarettes [65], which they might not otherwise have consumed. In other words, the premise is that they will smoke because they used these devices first.

The question is: Would all those who later smoked have done so without first using these devices? Some authors [65] propose alternative hypotheses to the gateway effect, suggesting that other individual and social factors play a more significant role than prior use of nicotine delivery devices. This is supported by the lack of correlation between the increase in their use and the absence of an increase in smoking prevalence rates within these age groups.

8. Conclusion

Nicotine, the main tobacco addictive compound, is not the cause of the diseases associated with tobacco use, according to substantial evidence. When isolated from combustible tobacco, nicotine presents a significantly lower risk profile than cigarettes and could play a pivotal role in tobacco control, similar to the contributions of nicotine replacement therapies (NRTs).

The emergence and development of new nicotine delivery devices, such as electronic cigarettes, heated tobacco products, and nicotine pouches, have transformed the landscape of tobacco control policies by offering alternatives to conventional cigarettes. These devices provide a pathway for harm reduction strategies, where the goal is not to eliminate nicotine use but to significantly reduce the harm associated with conventional tobacco consumption.

Although not risk-free, these devices are positioned as a less harmful alternative to combustible tobacco. By eliminating or reducing combustion, they significantly decrease exposure to harmful compounds. Moreover, these products offer a more acceptable and flexible way to administer nicotine compared to traditional NRTs, improving adherence to their use. Unlike traditional NRTs, they align more closely with the preferences of many smokers.

Additionally, these alternatives may contribute to the denormalization of smoking by providing options for smokers who cannot or do not wish to completely quit nicotine—but want to quit tobacco. This perspective aligns with the harm minimization approach, where the goal is not necessarily to eliminate nicotine exposure but to reduce the risks associated with its use.

In conclusion, a global perspective is needed to enable a balanced approach to promoting and regulating these devices, given the wide variability in global regulations. To maximize their potential, it is essential to strike a balance between encouraging their use as lower-risk alternatives—acknowledging that zero risk is rare in medicine—and implementing joint policies to prevent undesirable outcomes, such as youth initiation or dual use.

The harm reduction approach should not be seen as abandoning efforts to eliminate smoking but as a complementary strategy for those who cannot quit smoking through conventional methods. Modern devices offer a unique opportunity to address disparities in tobacco control by providing options for populations with high smoking rates. We must dissociate tobacco from nicotine use as a strategy and stop equating nicotine with the harmfulness of conventional cigarettes.

Author details

Josep M. Ramon-Torrell
Clinical Science Department, School of Medicine and Health Sciences, University of Barcelona, Catalonia, Spain

*Address all correspondence to: jmramon@ub.edu

References

[1] Organización Mundial de la Salud. Tabaco [Internet]. OMS; 2020. Available from: https://www.who.int/es/news-room/fact-sheets/detail/tobacco [Accessed: 8 October 2024]

[2] US Department of Health and Human Services. The Health Consequences of Smoking: A Report of the Surgeon General. Washington, DC: US Government Printing Office; 2004

[3] American Cancer Society. Cancer Facts & Figures 2020. Atlanta: American Cancer Society; 2020

[4] National Cancer Institute. Smoking and Cancer [Internet]. 2020. Available from: https://www.cancer.gov/about-cancer/causes-prevention/risk/tobacco [Accessed: 8 October 2024]

[5] GBD 2019 Tobacco Collaborators. Spatial, temporal, and demographic patterns in prevalence of smoking tobacco use and attributable disease burden in 204 countries and territories, 1990-2019: A systematic analysis from the global burden of disease study 2019. Lancet. 2021;**397**:2337-2360

[6] Hukkanen J, Jacob P, Benowitz NL. Metabolism and disposition kinetics of nicotine. Pharmacological Reviews. 2005;**57**(1):79-115. DOI: 10.1124/pr.57.1.3

[7] Russell MAH. The future of nicotine replacement. British Journal of Addiction. 1991;**86**:653-658

[8] Benowitz NL. Nicotine addiction. The New England Journal of Medicine. 2010;**362**(24):2295-2303. DOI: 10.1056/NEJMra0809890

[9] Changeux JP. Nicotine addiction and nicotinic receptors: Lessons from geneticallymodified mice. Nature Reviews. Neuroscience. 2010;**11**(6):389-401. DOI: 10.1038/nrn2849

[10] Mansvelder HD, McGehee DS. Cellular and synaptic mechanisms of nicotine addiction. Journal of Neurobiology. 2002;**53**(4):606-617. DOI: 10.1002/neu.10143

[11] Dani JA, De Biasi M. Mechanisms of nicotine addiction: Current understanding and future perspectives. Neuropharmacology. 2013;**76**(Pt B):529-541. DOI: 10.1016/j.neuropharm.2013.05.032

[12] Henningfield JE, Smith TT, Kleykamp BA, Fant RV, Donny EC. Nicotine self- administration research: The legacy of Steven R. Goldberg and implications for regulation, health policy, and research. Psychopharmacology. 2016;**233**:3829-3848

[13] Picciotto MR, Higley MJ, Mineur YS. Acetylcholine as a neuromodulator: Cholinergic signaling shapes nervous system function and behavior. Neuron. 2012;**76**:116-129

[14] McEwen A, West R, McRobbie H. Motives for smoking and their correlates in clients attending stop smoking treatment services. Nicotine & Tobacco Research. 2008;**10**(5):843-850. DOI: 10.1080/14622200802027132

[15] Hughes JR. Effects of abstinence from tobacco: Valid symptoms and time course. Nicotine & Tobacco Research. 2007;**9**(3):315-327. DOI: 10.1080/14622200701188919

[16] Albuquerque EX, Pereira EF, Alkondon M, Rogers SW. Mammalian nicotinic acetylcholine receptors: From

structure to function. Physiological Reviews. 2009;**89**(1):73-120. DOI: 10.1152/physrev.00015

[17] Changeux JP. The nicotinic acetylcholine receptor: The founding father of the pentameric ligand-gated ion channel superfamily. The Journal of Biological Chemistry. 2012;**287**(48):40207-40215. DOI: 10.1074/jbc.R112.404080

[18] Gotti C, Clementi F. Neuronal nicotinic receptors: From structure to pathology. Progress in Neurobiology. 2004;**74**(6):363-396. DOI: 10.1016/j.pneurobio.2004.09.006

[19] Lester HA, Dibas MI, Dahan DS, Leite JF, Dougherty DA. Cys-loop receptors: New twists and turns. Trends in Neurosciences. 2004;**27**(6):329-336. DOI: 10.1016/j.tins.2004.04.006

[20] De Biasi M, Salas R. Influence of neuronal nicotinic receptors over nicotine addiction and withdrawal. Experimental Biology and Medicine (Maywood, N.J.). 2008;**233**(8):917-929. DOI: 10.3181/0803-MR-47

[21] Koob GF, Volkow ND. Neurocircuitry of addiction. Neuropsychopharmacology. 2010;**35**(1):217-238. DOI: 10.1038/npp.2009.110

[22] Di Chiara G, Imperato A. Drugs abused by humans preferentially increase synaptic dopamine concentrations in the mesolimbic system of freely moving rats. Proceedings of the National Academy of Sciences of the United States of America. 1988;**85**(14):5274-5278. DOI: 10.1073/pnas.85.14.5274

[23] Rose JE, Levin ED. Inter-relationships between conditioned and primary reinforcement in the maintenance of cigarette smoking. British Journal of Addiction. 1991;**86**(5):605-609. DOI: 10.1111/j.1360-0443.1991.tb01817.x

[24] Ramström LM, Wikmans T. Mortality attributable to tobacco among men in Sweden and other European countries: An analysis of data in a WHO report. Tobacco Induced Diseases. 2014;**12**(1):14

[25] World Health Organization, editor. WHO Global Report on Trends in Prevalence of Tobacco Smoking 2000-2025. 2nd ed. Geneva: World Health Organization; 2018

[26] Foulds J, Ramström L, Burke M, Fagerström K. Effect of smokeless tobacco (snus) on smoking and public health in Sweden. Tobacco Control. 2003;**12**(4):349-359

[27] Talhout R, Schulz T, Florek E, van Benthem J, Wester P, Opperhuizen A. Hazardous compounds in tobacco smoke. International Journal of Environmental Research and Public Health. 2011;**8**(2):613-628

[28] Scherer G, Pluym N, Scherer M. Literature review on nicotine's role in human health. Tobacco & Nicotine Research. 2024;**33**(1):5-90

[29] Klein J, Diaba-Nuhoho GS, Brunssen G, Morawietz H. Regulation of endothelial function by cigarette smoke and next-generation tobacco and nicotine products. Pflugers Archiv-European Journal of Physiology. 2023;**475**:835-844

[30] Benowitz NL, Gourlay SG. Cardiovascular toxicity of nicotine: Implications for nicotine replacement therapy. Journal of the American College of Cardiology. 1997;**29**:1422-1431

[31] Ambrose JA, Barua RS. The pathophysiology of cigarette smoking and cardiovascular disease: An update.

Journal of the American College of Cardiology. 2004;**43**(10):1731-1737

[32] Scientific Committee on Health Environmental and Emerging Risks (SCHEER): Scientific Opinion on Electronic Cigarettes. Luxembourg; 2021

[33] Stratton K, Kwan LY, et al., editors. National Academies of Sciences Engineering and Medicine: Public Health Consequences of E-Cigarettes. Washington, DC, USA: National Academies Press; 2018. ISBN: 978-0-309-46834-3

[34] Glantz SA, Barecham DW. E-cigarettes use, effects on smoking, risk and policy implications. Annual Review of Public Health. 2018;**39**:28.1-28.21

[35] Gray N, Borland R. E-cigarettes and evidence-based policy: The importance of a precautionary principle. Cancer Prevention Research. 2018;**11**(9):545-547

[36] Hecht SS. Lung carcinogenesis by tobacco smoke. International Journal of Cancer. 2012;**131**(12):2724-2732

[37] Bekki K, Inaba Y, Uchiyama S, Kunugita N. Comparison of chemicals in mainstream smoke in heat-not-burn tobacco and combustion cigarettes. Journal of UOEH. 2017;**39**(3):201-207

[38] Dasgupta P, Rizwani W, Pillai S, Kinkade R, Kovacs M, Rastogi S, et al. Nicotine induces cell proliferation, invasion and epithelial-mesenchymal transition in a variety of human cancer cell lines. International Journal of Cancer. 2009;**124**(1):36-45

[39] Terzikhan N, Verhamme KMC, Hofman A, Stricker BH, Brusselle GG, Lahousse L. Prevalence and incidence of COPD in smokers and non-smokers: The Rotterdam study. European Journal of Epidemiology. 2016;**31**:785-792

[40] Andreozzi P, Gussoni G, Sesti G, Montano N, Pietrangelo A, The Italian Society of Internal Medicine (SIMI) Council Member Group. Impact of electronic cigarettes (e-cigs) and heat-not-burn/heated tobacco products (HnB/HTP) on asthma and chronic obstructive pulmonary disease: A viewpoint of the Italian Society of Internal Medicine. Internal and Emergency Medicine. 2024;**19**:1829-1837

[41] Moazed F, Chun L, Matthay MA, Calfee CS, Gotts JE. Assessment of the efficacy and toxicology of e-cigarettes. JAMA Internal Medicine. 2018;**178**(11):1546-1554

[42] Shields PG, Berman M, Brasky TM, Freudenheim JL, Mathe E, McElroy JP, et al. A review of pulmonary toxicity of electronic cigarettes in the context of smoking: A focus on inflammation. Cancer Epidemiology, Biomarkers & Prevention. 2017;**26**:1175-1191

[43] Chang CM, Cheng YC, Cho TM, Mishina EM, Del Valle-Pinero AY, van Bemmel DM, et al. Biomarkers of potential harm: Summary of an FDA-sponsored public workshop. Nicotine & Tobacco Research. 2019;**21**:3-13

[44] Morjaria JB, Campagna D, Caci G, O'Leary R, Polosa R. Health impact of e-cigarettes and heated tobacco products in chronic obstructive pulmonary disease: Current and emerging evidence. Expert Review of Respiratory Medicine. 2022;**16**(11-12):1213-1226

[45] Dinakar C, O'Connor GT. The health effects of electronic cigarettes. The New England Journal of Medicine. 2016;**375**:1372-1381

[46] Levy DT et al. Potential deaths averted in USA by replacing cigarettes with e-cigarettes. Tobacco Control. 2018;**27**(1):18-25

[47] Farsalinos KE et al. Safety evaluation and risk assessment of electronic cigarettes as tobacco cigarette substitutes: A systematic review. Therapeutic Advances in Drug Safety. 2014;**5**(2):67-86

[48] Sala M, Gotti C. Electronic nicotine delivery systems (ENDS): A convenient means of smoking? Pharmacological Research. 2023;**195**:106885

[49] Omaiye EE, Williams M, Bozhilov KN, Talbotv P. Design features and elemental/metal analysis of the atomizers in pod-style electronic cigarettes. PLoS One. 2021;**16**(3):e0248127

[50] Upadhyay S, Rahman M, Johanson G, Palmberg L, Ganguly K. Heated tobacco products: Insights into composition and toxicity. Toxics. 2023;**11**:667

[51] Leigh NJ et al. Cytotoxic effects of heated tobacco products. Tobacco Control. 2018;**27**(Suppl 1):s1-s5

[52] Hatsukami DK et al. Reduced nicotine content cigarettes: Smoke exposure and smoking behavior. JAMA. 2018;**320**(1):88-89

[53] Hartmann-Boyce J, McRobbie H, Lindson N, et al. Electronic cigarettes for smoking cessation. Cochrane Database of Systematic Reviews. 2021;**4**(4):CD010216

[54] Lunell E, Fagerström K, Hughes JR. Nicotine pouches: A review of the evidence. Nicotine & Tobacco Research. 2022;**24**(3):287-296

[55] Lindson N, Butler AR, McRobbie H, Bullen C, Hajek P, Begh R, et al. Electronic cigarettes for smoking cessation. Cochrane Database of Systematic Reviews. 2024;**1**(1):CD010216

[56] Hajek P, Phillips-Waller A. A randomized trial of e-cigarettes versus nicotine-replacement therapy. The New England Journal of Medicine. 2019;**380**(7):629-637

[57] Caponnetto P, Campagna D, Papale G. The emerging phenomenon of heated tobacco products: A narrative review. Current Opinion in Psychology. 2020;**30**:77-83

[58] Tattan-Birch H, Hartmann-Boyce J, Kock L, Simonavicius E, Brose L, Jackson S, et al. Heated tobacco products for smoking cessation and reducing smoking prevalence. Cochrane Database of Systematic Reviews. 2022;**1**:CD013790

[59] Caponnetto P, Campagna D, Maglia M, Benfatto F, Emma R, Caruso M, et al. Comparing the effectiveness, tolerability, and acceptability of heated tobacco products and refillable electronic cigarettes for cigarette substitution (CEASEFIRE): Randomized controlled trial. JMIR Public Health and Surveillance. 2023;**9**:e42628

[60] Royal College of Physicians. Nicotine without Smoke: Tobacco Harm Reduction. London: RCP; 2016

[61] Shahab L, Goniewicz ML, Blount BC, et al. Nicotine, carcinogen, and toxin exposure in long-term E-cigarette and nicotine replacement therapy users: A cross-sectional study. Annals of Internal Medicine. 2017;**21**(166):350-400

[62] National Institute on Drug Abuse. Cigarrillos electrónicos (e-cigs)—DrugFacts. Available from: https://nida.nih.gov/es/publicaciones/drugfacts/cigarrillos-electronicos-e-cigs [Accessed: 3 January 2025]

[63] Soneji S, Barrington-Trimis JL, Wills TA, Leventhal AM, Unger JB, Gibson LA, et al. Association between initial use of e-cigarettes and subsequent cigarette smoking among adolescents and young adults: A systematic review and meta-analysis. JAMA Pediatrics. 2017;**171**(8):788-797

[64] National Academies of sciences engineering and medicine. In: Eaton DL, Kwan LY, Stratton K, editors. Public Health Consequences of E-Cigarettes. Washington (DC): National Academies Press; 2018

[65] Selya A. The "gateway" hypothesis: Evaluation of evidence and alternative explanations. Harm Reduction Journal. 2024;**21**:113

Chapter 5

Does Morphine Abuse Harm Male Reproductive System?

Zulfikare Isik Solak Gormus and Raviye Ozen Koca

Abstract

Opioids have been used for both medicinal and recreational purposes (abuse) since ancient times. One of the most important opioids is morphine, a natural alkaloid obtained from the poppy plant (*Papaver somniferum*). The word morphine comes from Greek Mythology, derived from the name of "Morpheus," known as the god of sleep in mythology. It is the most common opioid used to treat moderate to severe pain. Morphine is a mu opioid receptor agonist, and is a very powerful analgesic that also has affinity for other opioid receptors. Opioids are natural or semisynthetic compounds that have morphine-like effects. They are generally used as powerful analgesics in pain management. However, long-term use of opioids can lead to serious side effects such as addiction, respiratory depression, sedation, and sexual dysfunction. Studies on male reproductive system show that opioids suppress testosterone production and negatively affect gonadotropin secretion and spermatogenesis. The effect of opioids can inhibit the sperm production process in the testicles by reducing follicle stimulating hormone (FSH) and luteinizing hormone (LH) levels. Long-term use of opioids such as morphine can lead to decreased testicular weight, sperm count, and degeneration of testicular cells. Despite these effects, number of studies show that some physiological changes can be reversed after stopping opioid use. The effects of opioids on male reproductive system should be investigated in more detail and these side effects should be taken into account during the treatment process.

Keywords: morphine, opioid receptor, male, testis, abuse

1. Introduction

Opioid drugs are defined as any natural or semisynthetic derivative that has morphine-like effects. The term opioid has come into use due to the development of synthetic drugs and the discovery of substances that have morphine-like effects in the brain. The term "opioid" also includes opioid receptor agonists and antagonists, as well as endogenous opioid peptides such as enkephalins, dynorphins, and endorphins that bind to the same receptors [1]. Opioids are powerful and systemically effective analgesics used for both chronic and acute pain treatment. Despite their use in pain treatment, they have very serious side effects. Some of these are sedation, respiratory depression, addiction, sleep disorders, and sexual dysfunction [2].

Opioid substances stimulate receptors, which belong to G protein-coupled receptor (GPCR) family and are normally activated by endogenous opioid peptides. These opioid receptors are μ, κ, δ receptors. While all opioid receptors are promising drug targets for different aspects of pain and mood, μ receptors are unique receptors that can be activated by opioids such as morphine to induce potent analgesia. μ receptor agonists prescribed for pain management include fentanyl and morphine. μ receptor-targeted opioids are the most clinically effective analgesics usable, but they also have the potential to cause addiction [3].

2. Opioid receptors

Opioid receptors are found in both peripheral and central nervous systems [4]. In addition to its analgesic effect caused by the activation of opioid receptors, many side effects such as respiratory depression, inhibition of gastrointestinal transit, and effects on anxiety may occur. Agonists for μ or δ receptors produce analgesic and rewarding effects, while κ receptors agonists are dysphoric. Morphine and similar opioids are frequently used in treatment of chronic pain. In most patients, a decrease in analgesic effects is observed with the development of physiological tolerance during long-term drug use. Besides physiological tolerance, physiological dependence may also occur. This situation may cause the dose of the drug to be increased in some patients to avoid development of opioid withdrawal symptoms. To understand these complex physiological mechanisms, animal models of tolerance and dependence have been developed [5].

2.1 μ receptor (Mu, MOR)

μ receptor was the first opioid receptor to be discovered. It triggers euphoria and plays an important role in stimulating the reward center [6]. This receptor is found throughout the central nervous system in sensory and motor areas, including regions involved in the integration and perception of these sensations, such as cerebral cortex and amygdala. μ receptor subtype plays a critical role in opioid addiction [7]. μ receptors are most abundant in caudate putamen, located presynaptically on principal afferent neurons in the spinal cord, where they inhibit glutamate release and thus the transmission of nociceptive stimuli from A and C delta fibers.

The periaqueductal gray area is an important area for central control of nociceptive pain transmission. The periaqueductal gray area has a high distribution of μ receptors. It is known that the analgesic effect of some opioids is mediated by inhibitory ɣ-amino butyric acid (GABA) in this region of the brain. GABA acts to reduce antinociceptive output from periaqueductal gray area [7]. The most important side effect of μ agonists is respiratory depression through decreased sensitivity of central and peripheral chemoreceptors to hypercapnia. μ receptor agonists also have gastrointestinal side effects. They have an inhibitory effect on gastrointestinal secretions and peristalsis. μ receptor activation can also affect cardiovascular system, immune function, hormone secretion, and thermoregulation. μ receptors located in the intestines are responsible for gastrointestinal evacuation and secretion. μ receptor agonists inhibit gastric emptying by reducing peristalsis. This is the most prominent side effect of morphine and other opioid drugs [5, 7].

2.2 δ receptor (delta, DOR)

It is less widely distributed than other opioid receptors. It is found in the highest density in cerebral cortex, olfactory bulb, caudate putamen, and nucleus accumbens. δ receptors are located presynaptically on primary afferents to inhibit neurotransmitter release. These receptors participate in the analgesic effects of some opioids through both spinal and supraspinal regions. However, it has been determined that δ receptor agonists reduce gastrointestinal system motility and cause respiratory depression. In some experiments with mice lacking δ receptors, excessive locomotor activity was observed, and it was observed that this receptor could reduce locomotor activity under some conditions. In addition, anxiety and depression-like behaviors were observed in these mice and it was thought that it may be possible to regulate mood *via* δ receptor [7, 8].

2.3 κ receptor (kappa, KOR)

Another member of the opioid receptor family is the receptors called kappa or KOR. They are widely found in hypothalamus and periaductal gray area. Dynorphin binds to kappa receptor and creates a dysphoric and analgesic effect [6].

3. Morphine

Morphine is a natural alkaloid obtained from poppy plant (*Papaver somniferum*). The word morphine comes from Greek mythology. In this mythology, it is derived from the name Morpheus, known as the god of sleep. It is the most common opioid used to treat moderate to severe pain. Morphine is a weak base that is highly soluble under acidic conditions in water and poorly soluble at physiological pH in lipids (**Figure 1**) [9]. Although the medical use of morphine has decreased recently, it is known as the most powerful analgesic and pain-relieving agent [10]. Morphine is a μ receptor agonist, and all of the effects of morphine occur through this receptor. Morphine also has a weak affinity for κ and δ receptors and shows various effects through these receptors. After oral morphine administration, almost 100% is absorbed from the gastrointestinal system [9, 11].

4. Opioid dependence and withdrawal syndrome

Opioid addiction is a public health problem. Also known as substance addiction, this condition is a very serious chronic recurring disorder characterized by an increase in desire to seek and take the addicted substance when individual's access to drug or substance is denied, loss of control at the limit of intake, and the emergence

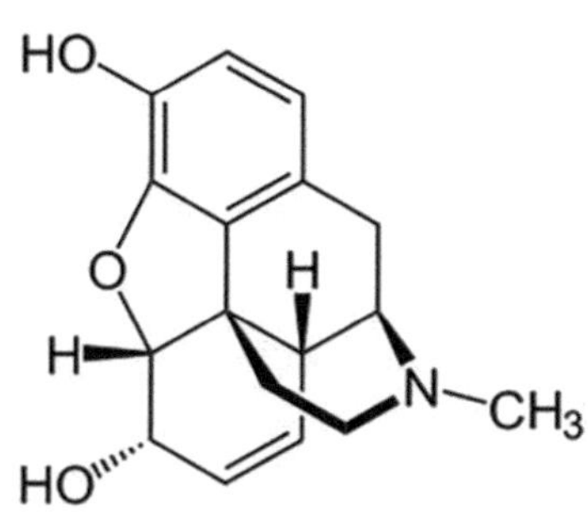

Figure 1.
Structural formula of morphine.

of negative mood states. According to Diagnostic and Statistical Manual of Mental Disorders (DSM-5), substance addiction disorders are defined as a cluster of symptoms including development of tolerance, withdrawal, uncontrolled increased intake, and craving for a substance [12].

Although opioid drugs have different mechanisms of action, all opioid drugs have been shown to activate the mesolimbic dopamine system. It has been shown that substances of abuse release more dopamine in these pathways than natural rewards and have a longer release time [13]. The basis of morphine addiction is how the brain's reward system changes as addiction develops. The mesocorticolimbic-dopamine system has been central to research on the neurobiology of the positive reinforcement effects of drugs. Opioids, and morphine, the most addictive form, inhibit GABAergic inhibition in the ventral tegmental area, which has a high density of μ-opioid receptors, causing dopamine release. Overstimulation of dopamine causes dysregulation of brain's natural reward pathways and learning processes, and development of sensitization and tolerance [14].

Opioid antagonists, such as naloxone, reverse the effects of opioid overdose by inhibiting μ-opioid receptor. μ-opioid receptor inhibition causes acute withdrawal symptoms in opioid addicts. μ-opioid receptor antagonists are commonly used in rapid detoxification to facilitate transition from addiction to abstinence. Since μ-opioid receptor blockade results in decreased efficacy of administered opioids, it can also be used to prevent relapse of symptoms [15]. Naloxone is widely used to prevent the effects of opioid overdose. Half-life of naloxone is approximately 30 minutes, which is considerably shorter than that of opioids. Therefore, respiratory distress caused by opioids may return after the effects of naloxone wear off [16].

5. Opioid effects on male reproductive system

While opioid addiction has always been a serious problem, it has recently become a global problem. Morphine addiction and withdrawal syndrome have many negative effects on human health.

Morphine and reproductive system studies have a long history. In the mid-70s, electrical stimulation studies were conducted on the muscles of experimental animals. It was determined that morphine prevented electrically stimulated contractions of longitudinal muscle of mouse vas deferens. This effect was stereospecific, and it was also determined that it could be antagonized *via* naloxone or naltrexone [17].

Opioid use disorder causes many different effects, most of which have been investigated in the central nervous system. Its role in reproductive system and testicular functions has also been investigated in many studies. Plasma testosterone, loss of libido, decreased ejaculate volume, and decreased sperm motility have been found to be associated with heroin and methadone [18, 19]. In recent years, efforts have been made to interfere with the complex network of opioid signaling at the molecular level, aiming to preserve analgesic effects while reducing the serious side effects associated with opioid use [20].

Some studies have revealed that motor activity of testicular capsule plays a role in the transport of sperm from seminiferous tubules to caput epididymis, in maintaining testicular interstitial pressure and in controlling testicular blood flow [21]. Opioid receptors are found in many places in our body. They are also located in many different places in the reproductive system, and endogenous opioids are found in different testicular cells.

The existence of three types of opioid receptors in rat testes has been proven. There are many studies showing its presence in Sertoli cells, spermatozoa, and Leydig cells [22, 23]. In addition the presence of μ, δ and κ receptors in the human sperm membrane have been reported. It has been also recorded that μ, δ, and κ opioid receptors are found in spermatogenic cells [24].

In a human study, the expression of μ receptors in sperm cells was investigated *via* immunoblot and immunocytochemistry analyses. The results showed that receptor was localized in the acrosomal region and the neck of sperm head. These results suggest a possible role for the μ receptors in mediating the effects of endogenous opioid peptides on sperm cells during complex and poorly characterized cellular events that enable spermatozoa to fertilize oocytes [25].

Infertility is a significant problem affecting a considerable number of couples of reproductive age. It is generally estimated that the main cause of infertility is the male partner. Genetic diseases, injuries, anatomical defects, low sperm count, and hormonal disorders can be considered as the main causes. The opioid system shows its effects through many hormones. FSH and LH act directly on the testicles and stimulate somatic cells that contribute to spermatogenesis. The synthesis and release of FSH and LH are controlled by gonadotropin-releasing hormone secreted from hypothalamus. The main function of FSH is to stimulate the proliferation of Sertoli cells during puberty, while LH regulates testosterone synthesis in adult testes. While the use or administration of morphine is associated with the suppression of LH release from these hormones, opioid antagonists such as naloxone and naltrexone cause an increase in serum LH levels in humans and many animal species [26].

It is known that Sertoli and Leydig cells of testis are affected by the local opioid system. LH and corticotropin-releasing factor also stimulate the production of endogenous opioid peptides from Leydig cells. Opioids may indirectly affect testosterone levels by inhibiting the production of androgen-binding protein. Endogenous opioids can exert an inhibitory effect on Sertoli cells, which provide metabolic support for germ cell differentiation [27, 28].

Opioids generally reduce not only LH but also testosterone and estradiol, which have effects on testicular function [29]. In fact, opioid abuse primarily leads to hypogonadism, including decreased libido and erectile dysfunction and infertility in men [30]. Administration of opioid antagonists such as naltrexone may improve symptoms of hypogonadism and erectile function, but antagonists do not increase testosterone or LH levels, suggesting a central rather than peripheral regulation [31]. The male reproductive system efficiency depends on regular functioning of a complex system consisting of many organs, the proper secretion of gonadotropes, and the cooperation of androgens and local hormones. It is essential for all these systems mentioned to function properly for spermatogenesis [32].

Opioids and their agonists reduce LH secretion in healthy men through a variety of effects on pulsatile gonadotropin-releasing hormone secretion. LH secretion decreases during continuous infusion of 5-alpha dihydrotestosterone, but LH secretion can return to baseline levels through an opioid receptor antagonist. FSH levels are known not to change significantly with opioid infusions. The effect of opioids has been shown to depend on puberty. This emphasizes the relationship between steroid sex hormones and opioid system. It has been reported that LH secretion in males increases in late adolescence under the influence of naloxone. Conversely, in the early stages of puberty, LH secretion has been noticed to decrease after administration of opioid antagonists [33–35]. Endogenous opioid peptides reduce testosterone production by inhibiting testosterone release and gonadotropin-releasing hormone. The effect of any opioid in terms of FSH levels was not determined [30].

Opioid and derivative drugs adversely affect male reproductive functions, including spermatogenesis, androgen capacity, sperm quality, and sexual drive. These drugs directly cause testicular toxicity by promoting ROS-induced testicular and sperm oxidative damage, inflammation, and apoptosis and also affect the hypothalamic-pituitary-testicular axis. This results in the suppression of circulating androgen, ruined spermatogenesis, and decreased sperm quality. Abuse of opioid drugs not only damages male sexual functions, namely, testosterone concentration, spermatogenesis, and sperm quality, but also alters testicular histoarchitecture through a series of events in multiple pathways [36].

6. Opioid effects on experimental models of male reproductive system

Results from numerous studies on effects of opioid use on the male reproductive system are associated with a significant decrease in the efficiency of sex hormones and spermatogenesis [29, 37, 38]. In addition to these effects, a significant decrease in LH levels in general, but no decrease in FSH and testosterone levels, has been shown [29]. As a result of these studies, it has been revealed that chronic opioid exposure causes some significant changes in sexual functions and sex hormones, but more detailed and meticulous studies are required.

Various studies have been conducted to evaluate addictive effects of morphine and morphine derivatives on rat spermatogenesis, and changes in spermatogenesis function were observed in opioid addicted rats. The population of spermatogonia, spermatocyte, spermatid, and spermatozoa stages in addicted rats was significantly reduced compared to the group not receiving opioids. Histological studies also supported this situation; it was revealed that changes in different opioid administration groups could affect sperm formation. It was determined that morphine in particular caused a decrease in sperm count and could affect all stages of spermatogenesis [37].

In an addiction study, male rats were given intraperitoneal morphine injections. After bilateral orchiepididymectomy, hormonal and histological evaluations were made. According to morphine-addicted group, sex hormone characteristics and spermatogenesis levels were significantly reduced compared to the control group. While there was no decrease in FSH and testosterone levels, there was a significant decrease in LH levels. When histological sections were examined, mature sperms were significantly reduced. Chronic use of opioids can lead to changes in sexual hormones and functions. Therefore, opioids have the potential to cause infertility. These changes may result from the direct effects of the drugs on the seminiferous tubules, their effects on the pituitary or hypothalamus, or both [39].

In a prospective experimental study, the administration of tramadol, an agonist to the μ opioid receptor, was examined for sex hormones, FSH, LH, and histopathological changes. Unlike other studies, FSH levels in the blood showed a significant decrease. In addition, degeneration occurred in the seminiferous tubules [40]. In another study examining the effect of long-term tramadol administration on testicular functions, a significant decrease occurred in plasma FSH, LH and testosterone levels, and sperm count. It also increased testicular nitric oxide (NO) and lipid peroxidation and decreased the activity of antioxidant enzymes [41]. Morphine administration decreased LH and testosterone concentrations and caused a significant decrease in testicular weight in a different experimental animal research. In addition, there was a significant decrease in spermatogenic cell population that governs spermatogenesis in morphine-treated testes. All observed effects were reversed within 13 weeks after discontinuation of the drug [42].

To evaluate the effects of morphine addiction on reproductive hormone levels and fertility-related markers, 30 male Wistar rats were administered two single daily doses of morphine intraperitoneally for 20 days. Male reproductive parameters (blood serum testosterone, LH, and FSH) and mRNA and protein expression of some genes, which play a role in fertility-related pathways, were evaluated using real-time polymerase chain reaction and western blot, and histological analysis was performed on testicular samples. LH and testosterone levels decreased, and expressions of all five target genes and target proteins were downregulated. By this study, it was concluded that morphine could reduce reproductive parameters in male rats [38].

Decreased libido is one of the major problems experienced by addicts. Erectile dysfunction has been reported in men using opioids for the treatment of heroin addiction. A study was conducted to investigate the effects of morphine addiction and detoxification with methadone on the male reproductive system as causes of sexual dysfunction in addiction. Serum testosterone levels, FSH, LH, testicular weights, partial weights of prostates, seminal vesicles, and seminal vesicle contents decreased in addicted group compared to the control group. In morphine-dependent animals detoxified with methadone, testosterone concentrations and seminal vesicle contents remained lower than the levels in control group. The results suggest that morphine addiction may impair reproductive function in male rats [43]. Low testosterone levels are characterized by fatigue, mood swings, erectile dysfunction, and decreased libido in men. This condition poses a significant obstacle to the treatment of opioid addicts [44].

Morphine is a psychoactive chemical substance that can negatively affect spermatogenesis by causing increased free radical production. So, what might be the effects of morphine use in men on sperm parameters, DNA integrity, and apoptosis? In a case-control study, sperm parameters (number, motility, and morphology) and sperm chromatin quality were compared with histological stains in samples taken from 30 men using morphine and 30 healthy men. According to data obtained from this study, sperm progression and motility in men with morphine addiction showed a significant decrease compared to the control group. In morphine abuse, it was observed that morphine reduced sperm chromatin condensation and increased sperm apoptosis rate. When these results are evaluated, it can be interpreted that morphine addiction may reduce male fertility by affecting sperm parameters [45].

Opium derivatives include morphine, heroin, and codeine; synthetic opium analogs include methadone, pethidine, meperidine, and so forth. Opioid addiction is usually treated with long-acting agonist opioids such as methadone and buprenorphine, which can affect the male reproductive system. It was investigated whether morphine detoxification with buprenorphine and methadone was related to male reproductive disorders in mice. Oral morphine addiction was induced in NMRI male mice (an outbred strain commonly used as controls in selection experiments and as experimental animals in biology, pharmacology, and toxicology), and then, detoxification programs were implemented using buprenorphine or methadone. According to the research results, number of Leydig cells and germinal epithelial thickness decreased after morphine use and significantly increased after detoxification with buprenorphine or methadone. Morphine altered oxidative stress, mitochondrial activity, and chromatin integrity in sperm, while detoxification with methadone improved mitochondrial activity but worsened chromatin integrity, whereas detoxification with buprenorphine did not improve either chromatin integrity or mitochondrial activity. The study reveals that long-term morphine use followed by detox with buprenorphine or methadone impairs testicular structure and sperm parameters [46].

The use of different types of opioids is known to cause sexual dysfunction. Testosterone levels were found to be higher in addicted individuals treated with buprenorphine compared to methadone. Therefore, opioid-mediated effects on steroid sex hormones and sexual function-behavior were seen in both chronic opioid users who need pain management and opioid addicts [47, 48].

Chronic morphine use has harmful effects on testicular function through the activation of inflammatory, oxidative, and apoptosis biomarkers mediated by suppression of somatic cells such as germ cells and Sertoli cells. Whether the deleterious effects of morphine dependence are reversed by spontaneous morphine withdrawal or incubation with methadone and/or naloxone in sertoli cells was investigated using an *in vitro* cell model of morphine dependence. CAMP levels were measured to assess morphine dependence in sertoli cells. Cell viability and inflammatory, oxidative, apoptosis, and glial-derived neurotrophic factor biomarkers were measured at the end of treatment following incubation of cells with methadone and naloxone and spontaneous withdrawal from morphine. Morphine dependence was shown to decrease cell viability and glial-derived neurotrophic factor levels and increase pro-inflammatory, prooxidant, and apoptotic biomarker levels in sertoli cells. Spontaneous withdrawal from morphine and naloxone was found to reduce pro-inflammatory and apoptotic biomarker levels in sertoli cells. It appears that morphine addiction increases apoptosis in sertoli cells, probably through oxidative stress and inflammation pathways [49].

When the effects of morphine and methadone on the endocrine control of sexual function in male rats were studied many years ago, it was shown that these narcotics caused a marked decrease in serum testosterone levels, which markedly reduced the structural and functional integrity of the secondary sex organs. Serum LH levels were undetectable in narcotic-treated animals, but serum FSH levels were unchanged. Based on these observations, it seems reasonable to conclude that narcotics inhibit LH secretion by an action on the hypothalamus or directly on the pituitary gland, resulting in a decrease in serum testosterone levels and a subsequent decrease in wet tissue weight and secretory activity of the secondary sex organs [19].

Opioid analgesics such as morphine and methadone are widely used to manage severe pain, but their potential for abuse and adverse effects on the brain and reproductive system are of concern. Their effects on spermatogenesis and cognitive function were investigated in male rats. Methadone and morphine were administered intraperitoneally. Long-term exposure to morphine and methadone resulted in memory impairment (short-term and long-term memory), chronic stress (anxiety and stress), hormonal disturbances (FSH, LH, testosterone, and estradiol levels), changes in gene expression (Tp53, CatSper1), and fertility complications. High doses of methadone reduced the number of offspring significantly. These effects were more pronounced at higher doses, emphasizing importance of careful dosing in opioid therapy [50].

It is already known that methadone is one of the most widely used methods in the treatment of opioid addiction. Although methadone is effective in the treatment of opioid addiction, sexual dysfunction and infertility have been reported as significant problems in patients receiving methadone treatment. The effects of melatonin and N-acetylcysteine on morphine and methadone-induced oxidative stress, apoptosis, suppression of blood sex hormones, deterioration in sperm parameters, and sexual dysfunction were evaluated in adult male Wistar albino rats. Exposure to morphine, methadone, and the shift of morphine to methadone caused testicular degeneration attributable to stress oxidative-induced apoptotic testicular cell death and impaired spermatogenesis. N-acetylcysteine and melatonin alone and especially in combination with each other improved testicular degeneration, testicular antioxidant capacity, sex hormone suppression, and testicular mechanism mediated by inhibition of apoptosis pathway. The study suggests that oral administration of antioxidants may be an effective treatment to alleviate some opioid-associated testicular degeneration and dysfunction [51].

Previous studies have shown that morphine negatively affects male fertility, while *Phoenix dactylifera* (dates) extract has been suggested to treat male infertility by exhibiting antagonistic effects. Thus, possible curative effects of dates on histological features of male rat reproductive organs caused by morphine addiction were investigated. In male Sprague Dawley rats treated with morphine, a honeycomb-like appearance with flattened columnar cells was not observed in seminal vesicle, while the absence of eosinophilic secretion from glandular lumens in the prostate gland was noted. *Phoenix dactylifera* administration improved the histoarchitecture of seminal vesicle and prostate gland with complex mucosal folds and glands with secretion-filled lumens. They claimed that *Phoenix dactylifera* extract has a protective effect against the negative effects of morphine on male rat reproductive systems [52].

Epigenetic marks can be affected by a variety of factors, including age, early life experiences, lifestyle, and exposure to drugs or chemicals such as "opioids." Previous studies have focused on how morphine epigenetically regulates different brain regions that play a role in dependence, tolerance, and other psychiatric disorders that are more related to pathophysiological effects of opioids. There is a wealth of information on the effects of chronic use on other organs and systems. A study was conducted on effects of chronic morphine exposure on DNA methylation and histone modification levels in individual organs of male and female mice. The results revealed that chronic morphine treatment caused systemic changes in DNA methylation/hydroxymethylation and histone modification *in vivo*, suggesting a potential physiological effect on regulation of gene expression. It is noteworthy that morphine-induced epigenetic modification is gender-dependent, suggesting different mechanisms underlying epigenetic modification in female and male mice [53].

7. Opioid effects on male urogenital system cancers

Recent studies have suggested agonism or antagonism of opioid receptors has important effects on cancer-related outcomes. Retrospective reviews suggest that increased perioperative opioid administration is associated with poorer survival in patients undergoing prostate or bladder cancer surgery for urogenital tract cancers, but the data are controversial. κ receptors have been implicated in both proliferation and inhibition of prostate cancer cell growth in *in vitro* studies. Similarly, the opioid growth factor receptor is highly expressed in prostate cancer cells and is suppressed by androgens. Prostate cancer tissue stains more intensely for mu opioid receptor. *In vitro*, opioid agonism induces urothelial cell carcinoma proliferation and invasion. Agonism of μ, δ, and κ receptors induces renal cell carcinoma tumorigenesis; opioid growth factor receptor agonism has the opposite effect on renal cell carcinoma. Evidence regarding the role of opioids and their receptors in urological malignancy is controversial. The effects of opioids on urogenital cancers require further investigation [54]. Preclinical studies suggest that opioids stimulate angiogenesis and tumor progression *via* the mu opioid receptor. Higher mu opioid receptor expression and greater opioid requirements are associated with shorter progression-free survival and overall survival in patients with metastatic prostate cancer [55].

Interestingly, opioid dependence can be observed frequently after urological cancers. In a study evaluatıng the risk of ratıonal opioid use after radical orchiectomy for testicular cancer. A total of 2911 men underwent radical orchiectomy for testicular cancer, and 89.8% of them were prescribed opioids at the time of orchiectomy. Patients prescribed postoperative opioids for orchiectomy had a statistically higher risk of developing new persistent opioid use. Postoperative opioid prescription after radical orchiectomy was found to be significantly associated with developing new persistent opioid use [56]. Castration resistance is a failure of prostate cancer therapy and is associated with ligand-independent activation of the androgen receptor. Loss of function of opioid kappa 1 receptor, which is upregulated in androgen deprivation, delayed the acquisition of castration resistance and prevented castration-resistant growth of prostate cancer both *in vitro* and *in vivo*. These data suggest that opioid kappa 1 receptor is involved in cellular adaptation to post-castration survival and castration-resistant progression of prostate cancer, accelerating the clinical application of opioid kappa 1 receptor-targeted therapy in the management of this deadly disease [57]. Opioids are preferred as a treatment option, especially for pain control. Metastatic prostate cancer may cause skeletal pathological fractures, bone surgery and/or radiation, and spinal cord compression. Opioids are frequently used in the treatment of skeletal pathologies. Long-term opioid use and dependence increase significantly after skeletal pathologies develop in metastatic prostate cancer [58].

8. Conclusion

Morphine is like a double-edged sword. While trying to benefit from its analgesic effect, it can cause undesirable effects on many systems of the body, such as the three-dimensional damage it causes to the male reproductive system.

Opioids, particularly those acting on the μ-opioid receptor, play a central role in both pain management and the development of addiction. However, their impact on the male reproductive system is concerning, with many studies showing that chronic opioid use can significantly impair reproductive health, reduce testosterone levels, and affect spermatogenesis by altering oxidative stress, mitochondrial activity, and chromatin integrity in sperm. These effects may be reversed to some extent after opioid discontinuation, but more research is needed to fully understand long-term consequences of opioid use on male reproductive health.

Author details

Zulfikare Isik Solak Gormus* and Raviye Ozen Koca
Necmettin Erbakan University School of Medicine, Konya, Turkey

*Address all correspondence to: igormus@gmail.com

References

[1] Koob GF, Arends MA, Le Moal M. Drugs, Addiction, and the Brain. 1st ed. Academic Press; 2014. eBook ISBN: 9780123869593, Hardback ISBN: 9780123869371

[2] Schuchat A, Houry D, Guy GP. New data on opioid use and prescribing in the United States. JAMA - Journal of the American Medical Association. 2017;**318**(5):425-426

[3] Ehrlich AT, Semache M, Gross F, et al. Biased signaling of the mu opioid receptor revealed in native neurons. iScience. 2019;**14**:47-57. DOI: 10.1016/j.isci.2019.03.011

[4] Waldhoer M, Bartlett SE, Whistler JL. Opioid receptors. Annual Review of Biochemistry. 2004;**73**:953-990

[5] Listos J, Łupina M, Talarek S, Mazur A, Orzelska-Górka J, Kotlińska J. The mechanisms involved in morphine addiction: An overview. International Journal of Molecular Sciences. 3 Sep 2019;**20**(17):4302. DOI: 10.3390/ijms20174302. PMID: 31484312; PMCID: PMC6747116

[6] Wang S. Historical review: Opiate addiction and opioid receptors. Cell Transplantation. 2019;**28**(3):233-238. DOI: 10.1177/0963689718811060

[7] McDonald J, Lambert DG. Opioid receptors. Continuing Education in Anaesthesia Critical Care & Pain. 2005;**5**(1):22-25

[8] Akil H, Owens C, Gutstein H, Taylor L, Curran E, Watson S. Endogenous opioids: Overview and current issues. Drug and Alcohol Dependence. 1998;**51**(1-2):127-140. DOI: 10.1016/s0376-8716(98)00071-4

[9] Sverrisdóttir E, Lund TM, Olesen AE, Drewes AM, Christrup LL, Kreilgaard M. A review of morphine and morphine-6-glucuronide's pharmacokinetic-pharmacodynamic relationships in experimental and clinical pain. European Journal of Pharmaceutical Sciences. 2015;**74**:45-62

[10] Bhatt K, Kumar A. Mechanism of morphine addiction by inhibiting the soluble Guanylate Cyclase-Nitric Oxide (sGC-NO) pathway. Mathematical Biosciences. 2015;**266**:85-92. DOI: 10.1016/j.mbs.2015.06.004

[11] Christrup LL. Morphine metabolites. Acta Anaesthesiologica Scandinavica. 1997;**41**(1 II):116-122

[12] Koob GF. A role for brain stress systems in addiction. Neuron. 2008;**59**(1):11-34

[13] Koob GF, Volkow ND. Neurocircuitry of addiction. Neuropsychopharmacology. 2010;**35**(1):217-238. DOI: 10.1038/npp.2009.110

[14] Uhlve GR, Koob GF, Cable J, Kim S, Kwok S, Mayes LC, et al. The neurobiology of addiction. Annals of the New York Academy of Sciences. 2017;**714**(1):5-28. Available from: http://link.springer.com/10.1007/978-3-319-69535-8

[15] Fiellin DA, O'Connor PG. Clinical practice. Office-based treatment of opioid-dependent patients. The New England Journal of Medicine. 2002;**347**(11):817-823. DOI: 10.1056/NEJMcp013579

[16] van Dorp E, Yassen A, Dahan A. Naloxone treatment in opioid addiction:

The risks and benefits. Expert Opinion on Drug Safety. Mar 2007;**6**(2):125-132. DOI: 10.1517/14740338.6.2.125. PMID: 17367258

[17] Hughes J, Kosterlitz HW, Leslie FM. Effect of morphine on adrenergic transmission in the mouse vas deferens. Assessment of agonist and antogonist potencies of narcotic analgesics. British Journal of Pharmacology. 1975;**53**(3):371-381. DOI: 10.1111/j.1476-5381.1975.tb07373.x

[18] Cicero TJ, Bell RD, Wiest WG, Allison JH, Polakoski K, Robins E. Function of the male sex organs in heroin and methadone users. The New England Journal of Medicine. 1975;**296**:882-887

[19] Mendelson JH, Mendelson JE, Patch VD. Plasma testosterone levels in heroin addiction and during methadone maintenance. The Journal of Pharmacology and Experimental Therapeutics. 1975;**192**:211-217

[20] Basaran MB, Koca RO, Gormus ZIS. Therapeutic innovations against opioid tolerance and addiction. Current Behavioral Neuroscience Reports. 2024;**11**:201-210. DOI: 10.1007/s40473-024-00277-8

[21] Setchell BP, Breed WG. In: Neill JD, editor. Knobil and Neill's Physiology of Reproduction. 3rd ed. Elsevier; 2005. ISBN: 9780080535272

[22] Ceccarelli I, De Padova AM, Fiorenzani P, Massafra C, Aloisi AM. Single opioid administration modifies gonadal steroids in both the CNS and plasma of male rats. Neuroscience. 2006;**140**(3):929-937. DOI: 10.1016/j.neuroscience.2006.02.044

[23] Babaei H, Sepehri G, Kheirandish R, Abshenas J, Monshi M. The effects of long-term administration of F on blood testosterone level and morphometrical and histopathological changes of mouse testis. Comparative Clinical Pathology. 2012;**21**:1527-1532

[24] Estomba H, Muñoa-Hoyos I, Gianzo M, Urizar-Arenaza I, Casis L, Irazusta J, et al. Expression and localization of opioid receptors in male germ cells and the implication for mouse spermatogenesis. PLoS ONE. 2016;**11**(3):1-16

[25] Albrizio M, Guaricci AC, Calamita G, Zarrilli A, Minoia P. Expression and immunolocalization of the mu-opioid receptor in human sperm cells. Fertility and Sterility. 2006;**86**(6):1776-1779. DOI: 10.1016/j.fertnstert.2006.04.037. Epub 2006 Sep 27

[26] Subirán N, Casis L, Irazusta J. Regulation of male fertility by the opioid system. Molecular Medicine. 2011;**17**(7-8):846-853. DOI: 10.2119/molmed.2010.00268. Epub 2011 Mar 16

[27] Almela P, Navarro-Zaragoza J, García-Carmona JA, Mora L, Hidalgo J, Milanés MV, et al. Role of corticotropin-releasing factor (CRF) receptor-1 on the catecholaminergic response to morphine withdrawal in the nucleus accumbens (NAc). PLoS One. 2012;**7**(10):e47089. DOI: 10.1371/journal.pone.0047089

[28] Seeber B, Böttcher B, D'Costa E, Wildt L. Opioids and reproduction. Vitamins and Hormones. 2019;**111**:247-279

[29] Bliesener N, Albrecht S, Schwager A, Weckbecker K, Lichtermann D, Klingmüller D. Plasma testosterone and sexual function in men receiving buprenorphine maintenance for opioid dependence. The Journal of Clinical Endocrinology and Metabolism. 2005;**90**(1):203-206. DOI: 10.1210/jc.2004-0929. Epub 2004 Oct 13

[30] Vuong C, Van Uum SH, O'Dell LE, Lutfy K, Friedman TC. The effects of opioids and opioid analogs on animal and human endocrine systems. Endocrine Reviews. 2010;**31**(1):98-132. DOI: 10.1210/er.2009-0009. Epub 2009 Nov 10

[31] Fabbri A, Jannini EA, Gnessi L, Moretti C, Ulisse S, Franzese A, et al. Endorphins in male impotence: Evidence for naltrexone stimulation of erectile activity in patient therapy. Psychoneuroendocrinology. 1989;**14**(1-2):103-111. DOI: 10.1016/0306-4530(89)90059-0

[32] Fard J, Karami M, Jalali NM. Interaction of sulpiride with morphine in induction of male rat infertility. Journal of Basic and Clinical Pathophysiology. 2019;**7**(2):6-11. DOI: 10.22070/jbcp.2019.4722.1120

[33] Delitala G, Giusti M, Mazzocchi G, Granziera L, Tarditi W, Giordano G. Participation of endogenous opiates in regulation of the hypothalamic-pituitary-testicular axis in normal men. The Journal of Clinical Endocrinology and Metabolism. 1983;**57**(6):1277-1281

[34] Delitala G, Grossman A, Besser M. Differential effects of opiate peptides and alkaloids on anterior pituitary hormone secretion. Neuroendocrinology. 1983;**37**:275-279. DOI: 10.1159/000123558

[35] Mauras N, Veldhuis JD, Rogol AD. Role of endogenous opiates in pubertal maturation: Opposing actions of naltrexone in prepubertal and late pubertal boys. The Journal of Clinical Endocrinology and Metabolism. 1986;**62**(6):1256-1263. DOI: 10.1210/jcem-62-6-1256

[36] Hamed MA, Ekundina VO, Akhigbe RE. Psychoactive drugs and male fertility: Impacts and mechanisms. Reproductive Biology and Endocrinology. 2023;**21**(1):69. DOI: 10.1186/s12958-023-01098-2

[37] Takzare N, Samizadeh E, Shoar S, Zolbin MM, Naderan M, Lashkari A, et al. Impacts of morphine addiction on spermatogenesis in rats. International Journal of Reproductive BioMedicine. 2016;**14**(5):303-308

[38] Ajdary M, Farzan S, Razavi Y, Arabdolatabadi A, Haghparast A. Effects of morphine on serum reproductive hormone levels and the expression of genes involved in fertility-related pathways in male rats. Iranian Journal of Pharmaceutical Research. 2021;**20**(1):153-164

[39] Ahmadnia H, Akhavan Rezayat A, Hoseyni M, Sharifi N, Khajedalooee M, Akhavan RA. Short-period influence of chronic morphine exposure on serum levels of sexual hormones and spermatogenesis in rats. Nephro-Urology Monthly. 2016;**8**(4):e38052. DOI: 10.5812/numonthly.38052

[40] Abdellatief RB, Elgamal DA, Mohamed EEM. Effects of chronic tramadol administration on testicular tissue in rats: An experimental study. Andrologia. 2015;**47**(6):674-679

[41] Ahmed MA, Kurkar A. Effects of opioid (tramadol) treatment on testicular functions in adult male rats: The role of nitric oxide and oxidative stress. Clinical and Experimental Pharmacology & Physiology. 2014;**41**(4):317-323

[42] James RW, Heywood R, Crook D. Effects of morphine sulphate on pituitary-testicular morphology of rats. Toxicology Letters. 1980;**7**(1):61-70

[43] Ghowsi M, Yousofvand N. Impact of morphine dependency and detoxification by methadone on male's rat reproductive

system. Iranian Journal of Reproductive Medicine. 2015;**13**(5):275-282

[44] Bawor M, Bami H, Dennis BB, Plater C, Worster A, Varenbut M, et al. Testosterone suppression in opioid users: A systematic review and meta-analysis. Drug and Alcohol Dependence. 2015;**149**:1-9

[45] Ghasemi-Esmailabad S, Talebi AH, Talebi AR, Amiri S, Moshrefi M, Pourentezari M. The effects of morphine abuse on sperm parameters, chromatin integrity and apoptosis in men. JBRA Assisted Reproduction. 2022;**26**(3):444-449. DOI: 10.5935/1518-0557.20210110

[46] Moinaddini F, Amirinejad M, Haghpanah T, Abedini M, Yoosefi F, Nematollahi-Mahani SN. Opioid replacement therapy with methadone or buprenorphine effects on male mice reproduction. Psychopharmacology. 2023;**240**(1):77-86. DOI: 10.1007/s00213-022-06274-7. Epub 2022 Nov 17

[47] Daniell HW. Hypogonadism in men consuming sustained-action oral opioids. The Journal of Pain. 2002;**3**(5):377-384

[48] Yee A, Danaee M, Loh HS, Sulaiman AH, Ng CG. Sexual dysfunction in heroin dependents: A comparison between methadone and buprenorphine maintenance treatment. PLoS ONE. 2016;**11**(1):1-12

[49] Pourhassanali N, Zarbakhsh S, Miladi-Gorji H. Morphine dependence and withdrawal-induced changes in mouse Sertoli cell (TM4) line: Evaluation of apoptotic, inflammatory and oxidative stress biomarkers. Reproductive Toxicology. 2021;**105**:175-183. DOI: 10.1016/j.reprotox.2021.09.004. Epub 2021 Sep 10

[50] Norioun H, Jamal Moshtaghian S, Alavian F, Khombi Shooshtari M, Alipour G, Ghiasvand S. Impact of chronic opioid on cognitive function and spermatogenesis in rat: An experimental study. International Journal of Reproductive BioMedicine. 2024;**22**(7):579-592. DOI: 10.18502/ijrm.v22i7.16971

[51] Mohammadi N, Shirian S, Gorji A, Roshanpajouh M, Ahmadi E, Nazari H, et al. The potential protective effect of melatonin and N-acetylcysteine alone and in combination on opioid-induced testicular dysfunction and degeneration in rat. Reproductive Toxicology. 2023;**120**:108453. DOI: 10.1016/j.reprotox.2023.108453. Epub 2023 Aug 2

[52] Baharin A, Hashim NE, Sonsudin F, Hashim NH. Morphine and Phoenix dactylifera (dates) effects on the histological features of male rat reproductive organs. Journal of Research in Medical Sciences : The Official Journal of Isfahan University of Medical Sciences. 2020;**25**:20. DOI: 10.4103/jrms.JRMS_681_16

[53] Muñoa-Hoyos I, Araolaza M, Urizar-Arenaza I, Gianzo M, Irazusta J, Subiran N. Sex dependent alteration of epigenetic marks after chronic morphine treatment in mice organs. Food and Chemical Toxicology. 2021;**152**:112200. DOI: 10.1016/j.fct.2021.112200. Epub 2021 Apr 21

[54] Lec PM, Lenis AT, Golla V, Brisbane W, Shuch B, Garraway IP, et al. The role of opioids and their receptors in urological malignancy: A review. The Journal of Urology. 2020;**204**(6):1150-1159. DOI: 10.1097/JU.0000000000001156. Epub 2020 Jun 9

[55] Zylla D, Gourley BL, Vang D, Jackson S, Boatman S, Lindgren B, et al. Opioid requirement, opioid receptor expression, and clinical outcomes in patients with advanced prostate

cancer. Cancer. 2013;**119**(23):4103-4110. DOI: 10.1002/cncr.28345. Epub 2013 Sep 16

[56] Alsyouf M, Farkouh A, Wood EL, Ghoreifi A, Douglawi A, Hofmann M, et al. Opioid prescription following radical orchiectomy associated with new persistent opioid use. Urologic Oncology. 2024;**42**(11):375.e15-375.e21. DOI: 10.1016/j.urolonc.2024.06.019. Epub 2024 Aug 3

[57] Makino Y, Kamiyama Y, Brown JB, Tanaka T, Murakami R, Teramoto Y, et al. Comprehensive genomics in androgen receptor-dependent castration-resistant prostate cancer identifies an adaptation pathway mediated by opioid receptor kappa 1. Communications Biology. 2022;**5**(1):299. DOI: 10.1038/s42003-022-03227-w. Erratum in: Communications Biology 2022; 5(1):718. DOI: 10.1038/s42003-022-03707-z

[58] Yaldo A, Wen L, Ogbonnaya A, Valderrama A, Kish J, Eaddy M, et al. Opioid use among metastatic prostate cancer patients with skeletal-related events. Clinical Therapeutics. 2016;**38**(8):1880-1889. DOI: 10.1016/j.clinthera.2016.06.018. Epub 2016 Jul 29

Chapter 6

The Physiological Functions of the Brain in People with Substance Use Disorder: A Systematic Review Using PRISMA

Matome M. Sekhotha, Pholoso V. Ngwana, Maanda Ravhutendele, Thabang O.L. Sekhotha and Onkgopotse O. Ntsoane

Abstract

One of the worst societal challenges affecting the world today is the development of condition of substance usage brought on by the administration of adulterated drugs. The administration of adulterated drugs mainly affected the central nervous system, specifically the brain. This is a mental health problem. The human brain may experience similar consequences from the usage of illicit drugs, like mental-related diseases. This publication sought to report the results that demonstrated the potential harm due to the administration of adulterated drugs to the physiological functioning of the brain. The technique for gathering data shall follow the recommendation for Preferred Reporting Items for Systematic Reviews and Meta-Analyses to form part of the results sections. These findings must explicitly show that those with substance use disorder (SUD) also have mental health problems. It should have been demonstrated by several writers that administering adulterated drugs may have detrimental effects on the morphology of the brain if the users do not seek medical help. One well-known serious adverse effect of inhalation of adulterated drugs is the development of spongiform leukoencephalopathy (HSLE), which can have disastrous consequences for the nervous system. According to an Amherst study, inhaling heroin significantly lowers the ratio of NAA to creatine in the hypothalamus. In contrast, the NAA/Cr ratio is thought to be a sign of neuronal density, total brain activity, and functional integrity. The current study's findings illustrate that using illegal drugs in any way has the potential to cause significant brain damage over time, which could result in death if expert medical assistance is not sought early.

Keywords: adulterated drugs, brain, cocaine, ecstasy, heroin, ketamine, MDMA, physiological functioning, substance use disorder

1. Introduction

Today, the development of substance use disorder (SUD) among people who administer adulterated drugs remains among the world's most pressing social issues [1]. Long-term administration of adulterated drugs may have a negative impact on the morphology and physiological processes of several bodily systems [2–4]. Cocaine and any other byproducts of opium production may be included as adulterated drugs. The European Monitoring Centre of Drugs and Drug Addiction is a crucial resource [5] that reported s that cocaine (COC) is the most widely used illegal stimulant, among young people. Adulterated medications are administered *via* snorting, intravenous injection (IV), or smoking-infused marijuana. As a result, a growing percentage of first-time young individuals SUD patients choose the snorting method rather than receiving an IV injection [5]. The effects of snorting heroin are felt rapidly, and although it is typically thought to be less dangerous than injecting heroin [6, 7]. The mucous lining of the nose and respiratory systems may be severely impaired or distressed if adulterated drugs are continuously administered through snorting [8, 9].

Administration of cocaine also has negative effects on the blood circulation and central nervous system [1, 10]. This is due to the fact that adulterated drugs are administered—by snorting or intravenously—that can have an impact on the central nervous system or the blood, respectively. Due to the various kinds of ingredients utilised in the production of these adulterated drugs, the detrimental effects on the central nervous system and blood may also affect other systems. The dealer uses different chemical ingredients to produce adulterated drugs [11]. It is standard practice to synthesise medications that are contaminated by using different pharmacologically chemical active ingredients that are only known to the dealer. These added 'adulterants' are said to make opioids more toxic and perhaps have new negative health consequences. The number of chemical compounds added is to increase the chemical components that make the contaminated product more toxic [12, 13]. The added ingredients may also increase the possibility of being more dangerous to the human body on their own. Unreported added chemical components are often included in these products to increase their benefits and encourage users to keep taking street cocktail drugs [11, 14, 15]. Nevertheless, these added components can be hazardous or prohibited, or their suitability for human use has not been thoroughly assessed. The additive ingredients are harmful and possibly synergistic effects of certain hazardous adulterants. They are then combined with illegally produced drugs of abuse that may cause overdoses [16, 17], serious health impacts [18, 19], and even death [20]. An addict uses drugs or engages in behaviours of administering repeatedly despite negative effects on health, unconstructive daily activities, deleterious relationships, and harmful societal responsibilities. Other people who suffer from substance use disorders often occur alongside disorders of the mind like anxiety [21, 22] and sadness [23]. Nyaope is a commonly used illegal substance in South Africa, especially among young people in previously disadvantaged areas [24, 25]. Users develop severe mental health problems and socially deleterious behaviour.

When adulterated drugs are administered, a cascade of chemical reactions in the central nervous system's millions of cells causes severe psychosocial behaviours [26–28]. Therefore, bodily chemical processes are influenced by these reactions. Receptors in the brain cells respond to chemical compounds of the adulterated drugs. Certain receptors only respond to specific kinds of substances. Opioid receptors are the type of receptors that respond to the administration of the chemical structures of adulterated drugs [24, 25, 29]. If a person suffers from SUD, the brain's opioid receptors influence human beings' perception of stress [30], pain [31], pleasure [32], despair [33], and anxiety [34]. They also have an impact on well-being, breathing [28], sleeping patterns [35], and eating [36]. Endorphins are substances that the brain naturally makes and binds to opioid receptors [37]. Endorphins help control body functions and lessen pain perception. Therefore, the chemical structures of the adulterated drugs mimic the endorphins and neurotransmitters. This mimicry allows these drugs to bind to the same receptors in the brain, leading to similar physiological effects [38, 39]. For example, opioid receptors in the brain respond to the chemical compounds found in adulterated drugs. These receptors are naturally designed to bind with endorphins, which are substances produced by the brain to help control body functions and lessen pain perception [40]. When adulterated drugs are administered, they can bind to these opioid receptors, mimicking the effects of endorphins and neurotransmitters.

Heroin's effects on the brain [41–43] can alter a user's emotions [21] and alter their way of life in a variety of ways. Knowing the effects heroin has on the brain can help someone stop taking the substance entirely. Therefore, if someone is currently using it, they should receive therapy by taking the proper steps. First, heroin depresses the central nervous system, just like other opioids and pharmaceutical drugs [44]. When heroin is administered, it is broken down into several molecules that bind to the brain's opioid receptors. Codeine and morphine, for example, function similarly [45] due to similar chemical structures. The human brain may experience the same effects from other substances that are abused. Cannabis administration may result in psychological effects, including a variety of behavioural patterns, as well as dysphoric reactions [46]. A person who administers amphetamine affects mainly the central nervous system, or the area of the brain that instructs nerves on how to carry out their functions, becomes more active due to the high production of dopamine [46]. Even though the human body system does manufacture some natural opioids on its own, the effects of using drugs and the administration of adulterated drugs are far worse.

Adulterated substances can change a person's reaction to pain, but they also increase feelings of pleasure and well-being by supplying dopamine to every part of the body, particularly the brain [45]. These extremely elevated dopamine levels may occur due to the effects of high elevated administration of adulterated drugs [47]. Then, how the medication is administered or how someone with substance use disorder SUD uses it. When opioid products are taken orally, the liver converts them to morphine before they reach the brain. When an adulterated drug is smoked, or snorted, it does not pass through the liver as compared to the administration through intravenous injection [48]. Adulterated drugs are delivered to the brain by IV roughly as quickly as smoking, which increases the drive to administer more. However, when heroin instantly reaches the brain [49]. Prior to attaching itself to the opioid receptors in the brain, it instantly degrades into morphine and other substances known as 3- and 6-monoacetylmorphine (MAM). A euphoric mood is created when morphine and similar substances attach to opioid [50–52].

The rewards pathways may be least affected by the repeated administration of opioid medications. The parts of the human brain that are impacted by the administration of opioid medications regulate the reward systems in the body. These could include the locus coeruleus [24], which is also responsible for creating dependence [53] and withdrawal symptoms [54], the frontal cortex [55], the nucleus accumbens [56], and the ventral tegmental region [57]. Long-term heroin use can alter the physiological functioning of the brain in a manner that can make it difficult to manage personal behaviour [58], process emotions [59], remember things [53], and make decisions [60]. Heroin use can have long-term impacts on the brain, such as impaired reasoning and problem-solving abilities, as well as trouble with social interactions and pre-planning. Therefore, the human brain can retain the modifications even after you stop using heroin, so you might still have drug cravings and challenges as well [61].

According to certain research, these alterations in the brain occur extremely quickly following the onset of long-term heroin users [28, 62, 63]. When the drug impairs judgement, a person may sustain additional kinds of damage. Moreover, those who have overdosed on heroin have been shown to have brain damage [64–66] or neurodegenerative [67] over time. Heroin slows down breathing; therefore, the lack of oxygen reaching the brain causes this type of brain damage rather than an overdose [67]. People must be aware of the significant brain damage that heroin can cause. Drug administration-induced SUD symptoms might appear rapidly and be difficult to reverse.

2. Aim

The aim of this research is to investigate the physiological effects of drug use on the brain in people with substance use disorders.

3. Objectives

This systematic review's objective is to evaluate and synthesise the results of earlier studies. The prior researchers ought to concentrate on the potential long-term consequences of administering tainted medications that could change the physiological function of the brain. Different keywords will be used to retrieve articles from the various search engines.

4. Methodology

To demonstrate how the brain is impacted in those with SUD, data was collected and synthesised using previously published articles.

5. Registration and protocol

The review was not registered.

6. Study selection

The keywords were first used to analyse the abstract. if the abstract passes the selection's first test. If the keywords were present in the material, particularly in the results sections, the article was downloaded. To make sure it tackles the intended issues, the piece will go through one more screening. The impact of drug delivery on the digestive system must be addressed in those matters. The methodology, findings, analysis, restrictions, and suggestions were reviewed and recorded. The primary focus will be on how administering adulterated drugs to individuals with SUD affects their brains. The findings, debate, and conclusion served as the foundation for the article's crucial point.

7. Eligibility criteria (inclusion and exclusion criteria)

The total of 37 studies were chosen for full assessment out of the more than 200 abstracts that were screened in order to ascertain whether all inclusion requirements were satisfied. Due to their failure to satisfy all of the inclusion criteria listed below, 16 studies were finally disqualified (**Figure A1**). Twenty-one papers were included in this review because they satisfied all inclusion requirements. The review was carried out by five researchers. In order to minimise inter-rater selection bias, a data extraction form was created to gather information from every research.

The study will include nearly all of the full-text publications that have been made since the inspection. Additionally, the research needs to fulfil the requirements given in **Table 1**. Articles that satisfied the requirements in **Table 2** were excluded. The publications were published in English and only appeared in peer-reviewed journals. Using comparable keyword sets, studies were taken out of each database.

No.	Inclusion criteria
i.	Relevant research that examined the effects of certain brain regions and the use of adulterated drugs
ii.	A title that is pertinent to the goals and objectives
iii.	Studies with ethical approval that use humans or animals
iv.	Examine information obtained from tertiary and/or research institutions.
v.	The study should use animal models or human beings
vi.	Studies published in English
vii.	The use of any adulterated illicit drug
viii.	The use of cannabis
ix.	Proof that the results were gathered using a methodology that was deemed appropriate
x.	Experimental studies
xi.	The use of magnetic resonance imaging
xii.	The findings from the post-mortem examination

Table 1.
An acceptable article was chosen to be featured in the results section using the information.

No.	Criteria
i.	The research projects that used prescription medications.
ii.	Study the used any unfamiliar drugs
iii.	Review articles
iv.	Participants that use alcohol

Table 2.
The following exclusion guidelines were used to be removed from the study.

Number	Heading used
i.	Year
ii.	Authors
iii.	Country
iv.	Sample size
v.	Participants
vi.	Type of adulterated drug
vii.	Statistical parameters
viii.	Method of administration
ix.	Outcomes
x	Affected organs

Table 3.
The following headings used to search for articles to be include or excluded in the study.

To complete the manuscript compilation, a last search was carried out from 1985 to 2025. Additional articles were discovered by applying a snowball method to those that met one or both of the requirements listed in **Table 3**.

8. Information source

The following search engines: Google Scholar, PubMed, Semantic Scholar, Science.gov, and Ref Seek were the first computer-based searches used to find the studies that would form part of this review. Abstracts from EBSCO and Science Direct were also looked up. To fill in the gaps in the information, we made an effort to contact the authors of any papers with ambiguous or unreported parameters, such as the kind of adulterated drug with an unidentified name. The time frame covered was 1985–2025 Medical meeting abstracts were excluded.

9. Search strategies

The following search engines were used to find the published articles: Google, PubMed, Semantic Scholar, Google Scholar, Science.gov, and Ref Seek [68]. The results section of the reviewed articles between 1985 and 2025, 250 were downloaded (Appendix I). The following keyword combination was used to select the relevant article: In order to obtain further information, such as publishing types and dates, any more related or common names were also used [11, 69]. The following keywords and the medical heading (MeSH) were used to build the search strategy: "Adulterated drugs," "Nyaope," "Heroin," "Crystal meth," "Methamphetamine," "Africa," "marijuana," "dagga," and "Cannabis" (Appendix II) in conjunction with the parts of the brain depicted in **Figure 1**.

At least two or three keyword combinations were tried to find the pertinent articles. As part of the articles that employed original research data, only 12 were found to be eligible for the study. Thus, in order to locate any publications that are pertinent to the current manuscripts. For the current manuscripts, we also used

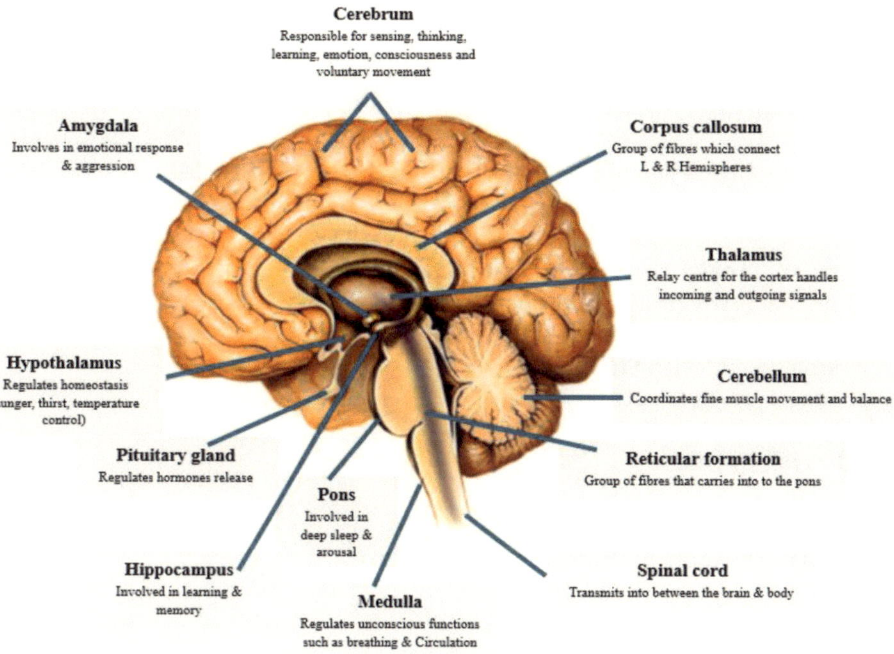

Figure 1.
The brain components [70].

forward and backward citation searches. As mentioned earlier, we also use authors to search many databases for forward and backward citations. We also used the University of Limpopo library's facilities to seek additional articles (Mr A Mothiba-Library assistance).

In order to filter the found articles, we modified the results section by utilising the records' title, abstract, and subject indexing. I then use those search phrases along with additional search terms I discovered during my inquiry to make a plan to find more articles. Furthermore, many search engines were used to locate and validate the search terms. The study was restricted to English-language publications and was designed to reflect South African rehabilitation facilities (**Table 1**); all 12 articles were found using various Google search engines (Appendix I). The number of articles used, the author or authors and the year of publication, the sample size, the type of substance being abused, the reason for using the substance, and the state of the rehabilitation centre are the variables that will determine the focus; these variables are presented in a tabular format.

10. Selection process

Various databases were searched for relevant literature using a general appraisal form for systematic review papers. A variety of subheadings were also utilised for the appraisal worksheet, such as the study's limitations, the year it was published, sample size, outcomes, and the goals, aim, and objectives for the type of substance being used. Using Mendeley and Micro Software reference manager, duplicate entries were removed.

11. Data collection

A structural form was made with the following details to make sure that pertinent data for this systematic review was gathered, as indicated in **Table 3**.

12. Data items

The current project's components were not categorised as originating from different regions. Thus, the findings will benefit the researchers because tainted medications, especially the novel and creative ones, eventually reduce the appetite for more drugs among people with SUD.

13. Study risk of bias

The Downs and Black instrument (Appendix III) was used to assess bias. To find reporting bias, the tool's multiple domains were used.

14. Results of individual synthesis

The outcomes of the manuscripts will be to inform the readers about the negative health effect of the brain due to the administration of adulterated drug. People who suffer from the development of substance use disorder (SUD). These types of behaviour may lead to modification of physiological functioning of the brain.

15. Biases in reporting

The possibility of bias among the studies that could affect the total quantity of evidence was assessed by looking at the recommendations made by the research. All included papers that complied with the same guidelines were included in the preparation of this review.

16. Features of the study

This will cover the kinds of studies that are carried out using either human or animal models.

17. Bias risk in research

The Downs and Black tool for evaluating bias risk was used for this (Appendix III).

18. Findings from individual research

Refer to **Table 3**.

19. Synthesis outcomes

Discussion compelled the results to be synthesised.

20. Results and discussion

The administration of most contaminated medications and other opioids, such as prescribed painkillers, depresses the central nervous system. Drugs that have been tampered with break down into several compounds that attach to opioid receptors in the brain [44]. Drugs like morphine and codeine work in the same way. Nevertheless, it pales in comparison to the effects of using medications like contaminated pharmaceuticals; the body of a human or animal model also produces natural opioids [45]. The use of adulterated medications alters your perception of pain and makes you feel better because they release a lot of dopamine into the body, which increases feelings of joy and well-being. Therefore, adulterated drugs all produce their highly selective effects at very low concentrations toward different body systems [46].

The euphoric effects produced by the administration of adulterated drugs is caused by these incredible productions of high quantities of dopamine [71–73]. The method of administration, or how you utilise the drug, determines how contaminated drugs react with your body. When adulterated drugs are administered orally, this may cause the substance to pass through the liver and change into morphine before it reaches the brain. When taken by injection, smoking, or snorting, the herb does not cross the liver [48]. Instead, the drug that has been tampered with enters the brain directly and immediately breaks down into morphine and other substances called 6-MAM and 3-MAM before attaching to the opioid receptors in the brain [74–76]. When morphine and similar drugs attach to opioid receptors, a dopamine surge occurs, giving users a euphoric high. Heroin affects the frontal cortex, nucleus accumbens, ventral tegmental area, and locus coeruleus, which is responsible for dependence and withdrawal symptoms. These areas are also responsible for controlling your reward systems.

In the accumbens and caudate, respectively, rewarding dosages of 1 mg/kg (s.c.) amphetamine and 5.0 mg/kg (s.c.) cocaine boost dopamine production and elevate the output of dihydrophenylacetic acid, homovanillic acid, and dopamine [77]. Dopamine is a key player in substance use disorders because it reinforces pleasurable feelings [78] and behaviours by associating positive experiences with a desire to repeat adulterated drugs overt a short period of time [79]. While 3,4-3,4—one of the byproducts of the neurotransmitter dopamine—is dihydroxyphenylacetic acid (DOPAC). One of the main catecholamine metabolites, homovanillic acid (HVA), is created when catechol-O-methyl transferase and monoamine oxidase operate sequentially on dopamine [80]. A reagent for identifying oxidative enzymes, homovanillic acid (HVA) is linked to dopamine levels in the brain. Brain and cerebrospinal fluid (CSF) fluid levels of HVA are assessed in psychiatry and neuroscience as a sign of metabolic stress resulting from 2-deoxy-D-glucose [81, 82]. The diagnosis of malignant pheochromocytoma and neuroblastoma is supported by the presence of HVA. The nucleus accumbens in the brain has several important functions and roles that include pleasure, dysregulation of depression, and modulation of limbic and motor systems. Hence, people who suffer from SUD develop behavioural patterns that are regulated by the nucleus accumbens by either high or low levels of production of dopamine and related neurotransmitters [81, 82].

In a study by Breiter et al., [83] 17 participants received cocaine injections while undergoing functional magnetic resonance imaging (fMRI) scans. Cocaine may increase the foci of signal change in many brain regions, according to the results section (see **Figure 1**). Craving and rush ratings were linked to the foci signal's formation. Therefore, there is a correlation between brain activation and rush rating, which has also been observed in a subset of brain regions, such as volume transmission (VT) and related organs, that have been linked to brain reward in animal trials [84]. Hence, the administration of cocaine between the control and experimental animals affected the physiological functioning of the brain over time. The affected areas in the brain will, in the long run, negatively contribute to the physiological function of the body parts [85] and lead to behavioural and lifestyle modifications [86, 87].

According to Keogh et al. [88], a computed tomography scan (CT) of the first patient, a 27-year-old man with spastic paraparesis and altered consciousness. It showed widespread symmetric low attenuation involving the cerebral white matter, internal capsule, brain stem, and cerebellum. Furthermore, they demonstrated that an MR imaging study revealed dramatically elevated signals in the corticospinal pathways, cerebral white matter, especially posteriorly, and cerebellar white matter and peduncles. Symmetric involvement in the white matter at magnetic resonance imaging (MRI) is an essential finding in patients with adult leukodystrophies because it is commonly associated with inherited disorders [89, 90]. On brain MRI scans, lesions—abnormalities in white matter—are typically visible as bright patches or areas. Accordingly, global functional decline [42], mood problems [50], gait abnormalities [91], cerebrovascular accidents [92, 93], and cognitive impairment [94, 95] are all linked to severe white matter lesions (WMLs). The three stages of heroin-induced TLE are myoclonic jerks and spastic paresis, softer speech and motor restlessness, and ataxia. The latter phase, which is marked by hypotonic paresis [96, 97] and spasms [90, 96], may be lethal [63]. The internal capsule's selective involvement of the posterior limb while sparing the subcortical white matter was noteworthy. After a seizure, the patient's condition gradually worsened, and he died six weeks after being admitted.

A study by Basch et al. [3] demonstrated that the histological examination showed diffuse reactive astrogliosis, microglial proliferation, and oedematous spongy myelin. The subcortical U fibres had not been impacted by the spongiosis, which involved the entire white matter. Considerable astrocytic hypertrophy and hyperplasia have been established by immunocytochemistry with anti-GFAP [98]. A few lipid-filled (Sudan Oil red-positive) macrophages were discovered intermittently inside the cerebral hemispheres' white matter. Most heroin abuse-related complications, such as rhabdomyolysis syndromes [99], peripheral nerve palsies [100], and immediate or delayed encephalopathies [90], have been linked to hypoxia [101], renal failure [90], arterial hypotension [101], trauma [102], and either explicit or controlled toxicology of both the substance in question or its contaminants.

A relatively rare, swiftly expanding, potentially fatal, and debilitating disorder that affects the white matter of the brain, namely the myelin sheath, is known as toxic leukoencephalopathy. It has been previously linked to being exposed to many leukotoxic offenders, including cranial radiation [103], chemotherapy [104], certain medications, and environmental variables [105]. These toxic-induced white matter degenerative results in the brain are becoming more common in the modern period because of the increase in the use of illegal drugs. In particular, white matter inflammation of the brain is distinguished by unique imaging and brain biopsy findings following heroin vapour inhalation [97, 106]. Similar results have been noted in the usage of cocaine [107] and other opioid products [108].

Heroin vapour inhalation, which has gained popularity among heroin addicts due to its ease of use and reduced risk of overdose, is closely linked to the rare illness known as "heroin-induced spongiform leukoencephalopathy" (HSLE). One condition that damages the brain's white matter is leukoencephalopathy [96, 97, 108]. The fatty covering that covers nerve cells, known as the myelin sheath, is defective in its development or upkeep. Leukoencephalopathies result in symptoms and indicators associated with disruption of the nervous system's fibre tracts, specifically spasticity, visual impairment associated with disruption of the visual pathways, and, as the illness progresses, cognitive deficits associated with disconnection of different cortical and subcortical regions. There are three stages in which heroin-induced leukoencephalopathy can present. The first stage includes apathy [90], cerebellar syndrome [109], soft (pseudobulbar) speech [96], and motor restlessness [91]. The next stage is intermediate and includes pyramidal tract and pseudobulbar signs, tremor, and choreoathetoid movements. The last stage, known as the terminal stage, is marked by stretching spasms, akinetic mutism, hypotonic paresis, central pyrexia, and death. There has been a reported death rate of 23% [107]. The system is primarily affected by spasticity, visual impairment caused by disruption of the visual pathways, and cognitive difficulties later in the disease due to disconnection of different cortical and subcortical regions.

Critical to the proper delivery of oxygen to brain tissue is its concentration, which is higher in arterial blood than in the extracellular space of the brain [110, 111]. This oxygen is necessary for the metabolic activity of brain cells. Because blood flow is strictly controlled and largely constant in healthy organisms under physiologically relevant circumstances, brain oxygen levels are therefore strongly correlated with blood flow. The amount of oxygen in the inhaled air and the effectiveness of respiratory activity control the amount of oxygen transferred from the external medium to the vessels in the lungs.

A physiological parameter that is sensitive to changes, respiration's efficiency increases during physiological [112] and behavioural activation [91] but decreases after sedative drug exposure [113, 114]. Changes in cerebral vascular tone, brain metabolism, and simultaneous variations in neuronal activity all significantly contribute to variations in brain oxygenation, even if respiration-dependent variations in blood oxygen content regulate oxygen entrance into brain tissue. Many studies indicate that oxygen entry is influenced by neural activity through variations in cerebral blood flow and cerebral vessel tone, even though gradient-dependent oxygen entry is the main mechanism governing oxygen levels in the brain's extracellular space [114]. The brain can acquire more oxygen before its heightened consumption during functional neural activation thanks to this gradient-independent neural process, which is typically understood in terms of neurovascular coupling. This helps to prevent any potential metabolic shortfall that could injure brain cells. Constant consumption of oxygen opposes the increased intake into the extracellular space of the brain, hence lowering the brain's oxygen levels. The levels of this chemical in brain tissue are also impacted by functional neuronal activation, which similarly increases oxygen consumption [93, 115]. It is often known that extracellular oxygen levels are the result of a delicate equilibrium between opposing and highly dynamic forces; yet, little is known about the physiological variations of this crucial homeostatic variable.

A powerful synthetic opioid, fentanyl is widely used in humans for both general anaesthesia [116] and pain [117]. As a recreational drug, fentanyl has gained popularity recently [118] and frequently combined with heroin [119]. Given that fentanyl is 20–50 times stronger than heroin [119], using it illegally can have serious health consequences, including the potential for overdose death [120, 121]. Fentanyl causes strong respiratory depression [122, 123] in addition to unconsciousness [124] and analgesia [125], a result that carries serious health hazards. While fentanyl administration for therapeutic purposes has been linked to respiratory depression and tissue hypoxia, its effects on brain oxygen levels at dosages appropriate for human consumption remain unclear.

According to a study by [126–128] stated that fentanyl can result in a rapid decrease in N-acetylcysteine (NAc) oxygen, which is followed by a gradual and prolonged rise in NAc glucose. Additional research has revealed that fentanyl causes comparable oxygen deficits in the basolateral amygdala [129], indicating that hypoxia in the brain might be a frequent problem. Therefore, it appears from the subcutaneous oxygen measurements that reduced blood oxygen levels as a result of drug-induced respiratory depression may be the cause of fentanyl-induced brain hypoxia [129]. According to other research, fentanyl caused biphasic variations in brain temperature [115, 130]. It also had effects on brain glucose [131] and oxygen [101, 130] that were comparable to those of heroin, although with some notable exceptions.

A direct comparison of the two medications should be done with caution because of their different potencies and pharmacokinetics. Heroin and fentanyl both inhibit breathing and result in brain hypoxia [132], which is followed by hyperglycemia [131]. Hyperglycaemia, in turn, can lead to further complications in brain function and metabolism. Understanding these mechanisms is crucial for developing effective treatment protocols for overdoses and managing the long-term effects of opioid use. The study by Kiyatkin [132] showed that fentanyl was more toxic than heroin.

According to recent data on opioid usage in South Africa, people of African descent use heroin at a rate of 12.8% [133], while the lifetime incidence of alcohol and drug dependency in the general population is 2.6% and 0.6%, respectively [134, 135]. In South Africa, nyaope, a street cocktail drug with a potent heroin basis, is one of the most widely used narcotics [11, 136]. Nyaope is administered by intravenous injection, snorting, or smoking [137]. Higher-grade heroin combined with other household chemicals is the active ingredient in nyaope [11, 15]. When heroin enters the brain, it rapidly binds to opioid receptors and changes into morphine [138]. Heroin users usually describe experiencing a "rush," or an uptick in pleasurable sensations. The release of lactate dehydrogenase (LDH) caused through elevated nyaope administration was shown to be time-dependent in **Table 4**, as demonstrated by the higher LDH levels at 5 μg/μL and 10 μg/μL as exposure duration increased from 1 h to 6 h to 24 h. Exposure to 5 μg/μL and 10 μg/μL of nyaope dramatically decreased Bax expression levels at both time periods, indicating apoptosis in the cells. The significance level at the 1-hour time point was $p < 0.001$ [11]. According to the author, the data presented in this study shows that nyaope has harmful effects. Cell viability of SH-SY5Y cells decreased in response to nyaope exposure in a concentration-dependent manner. The primary mechanism of cell death was necrosis, as demonstrated by the elevated LDH levels following nyaope exposure (≥5 μg/μL). The evidence supporting a nyaope-induced apoptotic form of cell death was less compelling, with conflicting results found for the markers (Bax/Bcl-2) under investigation [11].

No	Authors	Country	Sample size	Participants	Type of adulterated drug	Statistical parameters	Method of administration	Outcomes	Affected organs
1	Turski et al., [139]	Poland	48	Sprague Dawley	Morphine	p-value<0.05 between abstaining and treated animals	Injection	The apoptotic cells exhibit nuclear condensation, cell volume reduction, and cytoplasmic contraction.	hippocampal formation, thalamus, amygdala, olfactory cortex, substantia nigra and neocortex
2	Di Chiara and Imperato [77]	Italy	25	Male Sprague Dawley	Amphetamine and cocaine	Factor 5 and 10 at p value <0.05	Injection	• Increased synaptic dopamine concentrations	• Accumbens • Caudate
						Factor of 10		• Stimulated dopamine release	
						Factor of 3.5and 2.5 (P < 0.01).		• Cocaine increased synaptic dopamine concentrations	
								• Induced behavioural stimulation characterised by hypermotility and rearing.	
3	Breiter et al. [83]	Massachusetts	17	Human being	Cocaine	P value <10^{-5}	Infusion	Areas of the brain that displayed localised increases in BOLD activity when initial stages of euphoria Decreases in fMRI signal susceptibility artefact	The brainstem (pons), neocortical areas like the lateral prefrontal cortex, lateral temporal cortex, parietal cortex, and occipital cortex, caudate, putamen, thalamus, medial temporal, and paralimbic regions (hippocampus, parahippocampal gyrus, cingulate cortex, and insula), and putative brain reward circuitry (NAc/SCC, basal forebrain, and VT) cortex.

No	Authors	Country	Sample size	Participants	Type of adulterated drug	Statistical parameters	Method of administration	Outcomes	Affected organs
4	Keogh et al., [88]	Canada	3	Human being	Heroin vapour inhalation.	MR images	Inhaling	Enhanced signal symmetry	The corticospinal pathways, the cerebral white matter, especially posteriorly, and the cerebellar white matter and peduncles
5	Meyer et al. [140]	Amherst	6	Marmoset monkeys	MDMA (Ecstasy)	MRI	Inhaling	• Increases in blood oxygen level dependent (BOLD) signal	• Intensity in multiple brain areas
								• NAA/creatine ratio was significantly reduced	• Hypothalamus
6	Offiah and Hall [141]	Unite Kingdom	6	Human being	Heroin	MRI	Inhaling	Ataxia, nystagmus, spastic quadriparesis	Cerebellar WM midbrain, pons, medulla
7	Bach et al. [3]	Germany	1	Human being	Flupirtine, Alcohol and nicotine	Magnetic resonance imaging (MRI)	Inhaling	heroin spongiform leukoencephalopathy	Hemispheres of the cerebellum.
8	Wang et al. [142]	China	20	Human being	Heroin	Magnetic resonance imaging (MRI)	Inhaling	Significantly decreased	Grey matter density ((GMD) in right frontal (superior frontal gyrus and middle frontal gyrus), left cingulate (Posterior cingulate), and occipital (inferior occipital gyrus) brain regions
9	Wnag et al. [142]	China	21	Human	Ketamine addicts	MRI	Inhaling	• Degenerative lesion	• In the brainstem (midbrain)
								• Atrophic	• Basal prefrontal (gyrus rectus)
10	Solis et al. [143]	USA	24	Long-Evans rats	Fentanyl	basolateral amygdala	Injection	Decreased oxygen levels changes in glucose levels	• NAc • basolateral amygdala

No	Authors	Country	Sample size	Participants	Type of adulterated drug	Statistical parameters	Method of administration	Outcomes	Affected organs
11	Nirban et al. [137]	South Africa	300	Human	heroin		IV	The total participants, 49.3% suffered from at least one mental disorder (MI).	N/A
								The three most prevalent mental health diagnoses were post-traumatic stress disorder (PTSD) (17.7%), generalised anxiety disorder (26.0%), and previous Major Depressive Disorder (MDE) (34.0%).	
12	Kashyap et al. [144]	USA	1		Heroin		Inhalation	Leukoencephalopathy	• Cerebellum
									• White matter
13	Bosco et al. [145]	China	48	Sprague–Dawley (SD)	morphine		Intraperitoneally injected	• Apoptotic cells exhibit nuclear condensation, cytoplasmic contraction, and a decrease in cell volume. They also separated from the surrounding cells.	—
14	Daniels et al. [11]	South Africa		SH-S5Y cells	Nyaope			Cell death by apoptosis	

Table 4.
Different articles with their relevant outcomes on both the brain physiological functions.

According to a study by Boitor et al. [146], one of the most severe side effects following opioid treatment is respiratory depression (less than 8 to 10 breaths per minute). This adverse effect is caused by the interaction of opioids with the central nervous system (CNS), which leads to sleepiness, decreased respiratory drive, and upper airway obstruction, as shown in **Table 5** In a study by Dayyani et al. [150], a review of risk factors and trigger factors showed that 62% of patients had an opium addiction, while 32.6% of control participants did the same. The odds ratio for opium addiction was 3.3 (95% CI, 1.4–7.9), while the odds ratio for opium consumption throughout the risk period was 8.1 (95% CI, 2.2–30.1). Additionally, every participant who had used opium throughout the danger period also exhibited opium dependence. Following correction for other trigger factors and univariate analysis, the results showed an OR of 9.2 (95% CI, 1.4–34.7) for opium usage throughout the hazard period (**Table 5**). Opium addiction is linked to the incidence of rupture-induced subarachnoid haemorrhage (SAH) [154]; moreover, opium use during the risk period is linked to SAH. Only when a subarachnoid haemorrhage happens on its own is it regarded as a stroke.

This study is significant due to long-term (more than 6 months) opioid drug administration that places patients at risk for developing central apnoea, which is characterised by abnormal breathing patterns during sleep. Opioids can suppress respiration by altering the neurochemical activity in the brain stem [155, 156], which regulates autonomic bodily processes including heart rate and breathing. There is a wealth of research that suggests long-term changes in sleep caused by addictive substance use, which may differ from some or all of the short-term effects of the substance. Curiously, both central nervous system (CNS) stimulants and depressants have comparable long-term effects on sleep due to the administration of opioid medications over time [157].

Opium dependence has been found to impact carotid intima-media thickness (CIMT), a measure of atherosclerosis [158, 159]. Cerebrovascular disease may result from the carotid's unfavourable morphological alteration, which will restrict blood flow to the brain. Whereby vascular events can be predicted with high accuracy by abnormal CIMT results [158, 159]. By analysing cerebral blood flow changes in response to a vasodilatory stimulus like CO_2, cerebrovascular reactivity was determined as an additional marker of asymptomatic carotid artery stenosis. A study by [151, 160, 161] showed that an increase in carotid artery intima-media thickness (IMT) is linked to opium addiction.

Acute intracerebral haemorrhage (ICH) is a disorder in which a blood artery in the brain bursts, causing internal bleeding and necessitating immediate medical attention [162, 163]. The incidence of ICH was substantially higher in patients with opioid use disorder than in the control group (OR = 4.23, 95%, as seen in **Table 5**, CI: 2.42–7.35, p-value <0.001). Additionally, the study by Saadatnia et al. [147] demonstrated that compared to non-opioid users, opioid users have a higher risk of acquiring ICH. Opium use disorder patients had a higher risk of infratentorial haemorrhage (22% vs. 12%), OR = 2.13, 95% p-value: 0.038, CI: 1.06–4.28.

Selectively attaching itself to voltage-gated calcium channel alpha2delta subunits and blocking excitatory neurotransmitter release Glutamate, noradrenaline, and substance P may be among them. Pregabalin, a novel gamma-aminobutyric acid (GABA) analogue, increases GABA levels in neurones [164, 165]. As of right now, pregabalin is the 30th most prescribed drug in the United States. In **Table 5**, the authors in Ref. [166] demonstrated that patients with SUD-P had higher odds of CI even after adjusting for other significant clinical and sociodemographic

DOI: http://dx.doi.org/10.5772/intechopen.1010039

No	Authors	Country	Type of substance used	Sample size	Odd ratio	Confidence interval	Outcomes
1	Saadatnia et al. [147]	Iran	Opium	806	4.23	2.42–7.35	The development of intracerebral haemorrhage
2	Kar et al. [148]		Codeine Oral tramadol Combination Multiple drugs over time	328	3.82 6.34 0.29 11.16	1.86–7.86 2.71–14.85 0.14–0.61 3.86–32.22	Psychiatric comorbidities
3	Boitor et al. [146]	Canada	Naloxone	266	1.024 1.842	1.01–1.04 1.10–3.09	Development of opioids induced respiratory depression CNS Depression
4	Abdelghani et al. [149]	Egypt	Pregabalin	160	3.14 2.47 2.64	1.46–7.86 2.57–4.91 1.71–9.84	Suffer substance used disorder attributed to the pregabalin that is associated with cognitive impairment in the frontal lobe
5	Dayyani et al. [150]	Iran	Opium	93	9.2	2.4–34.7	The development of aneurysmal rupture
6	Hamziee-Moghadam et al. [151]	Iran	Opium	93	0.004 0.010	0.00–0.39 0.94–1.13	The development of carotid intima-media thickness The middle cerebral arterial
7	Barber et al. [152]	New Zealand	Cannabis	160	2.30	1.08–5.08	Increased risk of ischemic stroke
8	Walker et al. [153]	Utah	Opioid medications	60	15.4	1.6–145.5	Patients with sleep-disordered breathing who used chronic opioids

Table 5.
The physiological processes of the brain following the administration of several types of adulterated drugs are discussed in odd ratios in a number of articles.

factors. This was especially true in the areas of orientation (P = 0.03, OR: 2.6, 95% CI: 1.2–4.9), delayed recall (P = 0.007, OR: 3.1, 95% CI: 1.5–7.9), and total Montreal cognitive assessment MoCA scores (P = 0.01, OR: 2.6, 95% CI: 1.7–9.8). Among patients with SUD-P, CI was common (47%); compared to control people, SUD-P patients had a higher likelihood of having CI. A daily dosage of pregabalin was linked to deficits in language, abstraction, and naming. N-type Ca^{2+} channels, which are in charge of hippocampus-dependent memory and learning, can account for these deficiencies. Pregabalin reduces the release of neurotransmitters, especially in the hippocampus and cerebellum, by blocking depolarisation-dependent calcium influx, which causes [166].

According to Barber et al., [152], the study demonstrated a link between ischaemic stroke and transient ischaemic attack (TIA) with a lifestyle that included cannabis and tobacco use. Cerebral ischaemia that occurs after or within hours of cannabis use, as well as recurring instances of stroke and TIA following cannabis re-exposure, have alluded to a causative association with cannabis [167]. In research by Barber et al. [152], cannabis was found in urine drug tests in 25 out of 160 patients or 15.6% of the population. An elevated risk of ischaemic stroke/transient ischaemic attack was linked to cannabis usage in a logistic regression analysis that controlled for age, sex, and ethnicity (odds ratio, 2.30; 95% CI, 1.08–5.08). There is enough data to demonstrate that most people believe cannabis to have few major side effects. Multifocal intracranial artery stenosis [168, 169] and reversible cerebral vasoconstriction syndrome [170, 171] are two conditions that cannabis may cause. Additionally, long-term cannabis usage is linked to elevated cerebrovascular resistance [172].

21. The executive summary

This project intends to illustrate the danger of the administration of adulterated from different authors worldwide. The administration of adulterated drugs causes more severe in the brain and related organs. This makes the people who suffer from SUD not add value to society and need professional help to cease the administration of adulterated drugs.

22. Future research

The prevalence of administration is increasing at a very high rate worldwide. The current study is one of the few projects that showcase the danger of administering an adulterated drug. In South Africa, we have witnessed the increasing use of the street cocktail drug called nyaope. In other countries, there is emerging evidence that people use fentanyl for recreational purposes. There is a need to carry out research to illustrate the negative health effects of these drugs on the brain that might lead to death. People who have already developed a substance use disorder due to administration must be admitted to a well-managed rehabilitation centre. In South Africa, there are a few rehabilitation centres that assist people who suffer from SUD. But more centres are needed to help the youth with SUD.

23. Conclusion

Opioids, which include prescription medicines, also depress the central nervous system, including heroin. Herbs that bind to opioid receptors in the brain are produced when heroin is broken down. Overdosing has been demonstrated to be more likely when opioids are used concurrently with other CNS depressive medications, especially alcohol and benzodiazepines. Strong opiate cravings, reflected in a decreased capacity to stop using drugs even in the face of damage and unfavourable outcomes, are a hallmark of chronic heroin use disorder. The term "chronicity" refers to the repeated use of opioid medications, which can alter opioid-sensitive neurons' and neural networks' ability to function and may even be irreversible or difficult to reverse.

For instance, long-term mu receptor activation from opioid medications leads to neuro-adaptation. Chronic heroin exposure causes neuroadaptations not just in reward circuits but also in other brain systems, most notably in cognition and stress reactions. Significantly impacted are the cerebral cortex, hippocampus, and amygdala, as well as their links to the nucleus accumbens. Any "neuroadaptation" brought on by an excessive saliency (importance or value) of drug reward is referred to as cognitive maladaptation. Some instances of cognitive maladaptation in substance users that may be treated with cognitive therapy include high sensitivity to short-term rewards and preferential attention to drug-related.

As previously mentioned, there are several neuropsychological problems linked to opiate addiction, both during long-term usage and following periods of cessation. Research on the neuropsychology of long-term opioid users has revealed impairments in executive functioning, including deficiencies in decision-making, inhibitory control, strategic planning, and cognitive flexibility. Comparing the performance of healthy controls with that of individuals abstaining from opioids, polysubstance users, patients with head injuries, or those suffering from chronic pain, however, revealed no obvious deficiencies in other research. The body of research generally suggests that long-term opioid use impairs neuropsychological function to some degree and that these impairments differ from those observed in acute and sub-acute users. The prevalence of chronic heroin use disorder—which includes fatal overdoses—has escalated to epidemic levels. Furthermore, there is some evidence linking long-term heroin use to the development of neurodegeneration and toxic leukoencephalopathy, among other neurological problems.

Acknowledgements

A special thanks to the people who supported me through this journey. I am very grateful to have the support from the University of Limpopo for their support. Also, special thanks to Mr. Abram Mothiba at the University of Limpopo, who works in the library, for his endless support. I am very grateful for the words of wisdom from Ms. Kedibone "Njamme" Mpherwane and all the Physiology and Environmental health staff members. A special thanks to my two special daughters Naledi and Kholo, for their continuous support and love they showed when I was compiling this manuscript. To Rose Ntsoane and Omphile Ntsoane, thanks for the encouragement and support. I always pray in silent for God to provide me with the strength to wake up early and work on this manuscript all the time.

A. Appendix

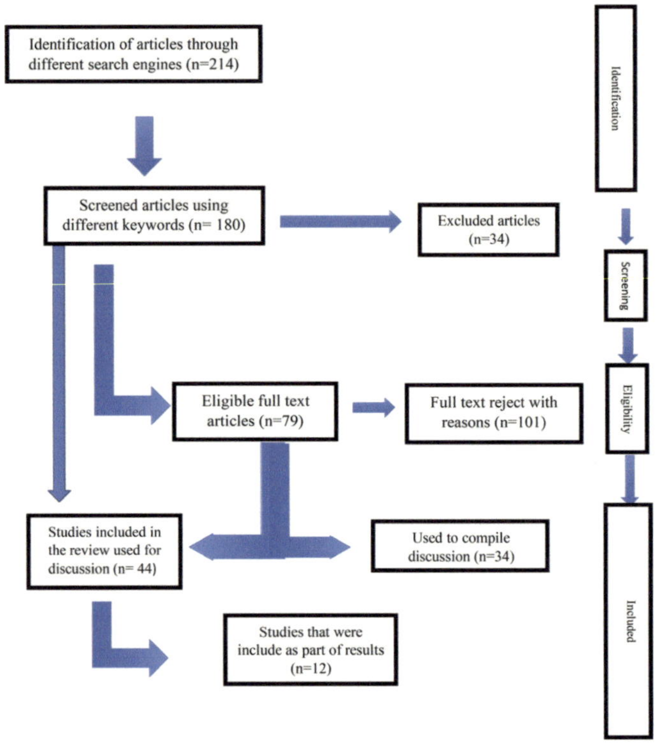

Figure A1.
Flow diagram to illustrate the searching strategy.

B. Appendix

See **Table B1**.

Search items	
Group 1: Adulterated drugs	
1	Cocaine
2	Crystal meth
3	Cannabis
4	Heroin
5	Methamphetamine
6	Nyaope
Group 2: Gastrointestinal (GIT)	
7	Various brain section as shown in **Figure 1**
Group 3: Target participants	
8	Rats

Search items	
9	Human being
10	Baboon
***Combining results**	
11	Group1 and/or Group 2 and /or Group 3 and /or Group 4

*The combination of groups will be done per items in each group e.g. 1 and/or 7 and/or 11 and/or 13

Table B1.
The search criteria for the existing literature.

C. Appendix

Modified Downs and Black checklist for assessment of methodological quality.

To assess the methodological quality of included studies, a critical appraisal was performed independently by two authors (IvR and SC) using a modified version of the Downs and Black checklist. In this version, question 27 is modified to whether a power analysis was performed (yes/no).[1] The maximum score was 28 and 25 points for randomised and non-randomised studies, respectively. A checklist specifically for uncontrolled studies that includes a scoring system could not be found. To facilitate comparisons, we used the Downs and Black checklist for both controlled and uncontrolled studies. Due to some questions (items 14, 15, 21–25, and 27) not being relevant for uncontrolled studies, the maximum score for uncontrolled studies was 20 points. In accordance with previous publications, studies were classified as excellent (26–28), good (20–25), fair (15–19), and poor (≤ 14) quality (**Table C1**) [173, 174].

Item	Criteria	Answers
Reporting		
1	*Is the hypothesis/aim/objective of the study clearly described?*	Yes = 1
2	*Are the main outcomes to be measured clearly described in the Introduction or Methods section?*	Yes = 1
3	*Are the characteristics of the patients included in the study clearly described?* In cohort studies and trials, inclusion and/or exclusion criteria should be given. In case–control studies, a case-definition and the source for controls should be given.	Yes = 1
4	*Are the interventions of interest clearly described?* Treatments and placebo (where relevant) that are to be compared should be clearly described.	Yes = 1
5	*Are the distributions of principal confounders in each group of subjects to be compared clearly described?* A list of principal confounders is provided.[a]	Partially = 1
6	*Are the main findings of the study clearly described?* Simple outcome data (including denominators and numerators) should be reported for all major findings so that the reader can check the major analyses and conclusions. (This question does not cover statistical tests which are considered below).	Yes = 1

Item	Criteria	Answers
Reporting		
7	*Does the study provide estimates of the random variability in the data for the main outcomes?* In non-normally distributed data, the interquartile range of results should be reported. In normally distributed data the standard error, standard deviation or confidence intervals should be reported. If the distribution of the data is not described, it must be assumed that the estimates used were appropriate and the question should be answered yes.[b]	No = 0
8	*Have all important adverse events that may be a consequence of the intervention been reported?* This should be answered yes if the study demonstrates that there was a comprehensive attempt to measure adverse events. (A list of possible adverse events is provided).	No = 0
9	*Have the characteristics of patients lost to follow-up been described?* This should be answered yes where there were no losses to follow-up or where losses to follow-up were so small that findings would be unaffected by their inclusion. This should be answered 'no' where a study does not report the number of patients lost to follow-up.	No = 0
10	*Have actual probability values been reported (e.g., 0.035 rather than < 0.05) for the main outcomes except where the probability value is less than 0.001?*[c]	No = 0
External validity		
11	*Were the subjects asked to participate in the study representative of the entire population from which they were recruited?* The study must identify the source population for patients and describe how the patients were selected. Patients would be representative if they comprised the entire source population, an unselected sample of consecutive patients, or a random sample. Random sampling is only feasible where a list of all members of the relevant population exists. Where a study does not report the proportion of the source population from which the patients are derived, the question should be answered as unable to determine.	Unable to determine = 0
12	*Were those subjects who were prepared to participate representative of the entire population from which they were recruited?* The proportion of those asked who agreed should be stated. Validation that the sample was representative would include demonstrating that the distribution of the main confounding factors was the same in the study sample and the source population.	No = 0
13	*Were the staff, places, and facilities where the patients were treated, representative of the treatment the majority of patients receive?* For the question to be answered yes, the study should demonstrate that the intervention was representative of that in use in the source population. The question should be answered no if, for example, the intervention was undertaken in a specialist centre that was unrepresentative of the hospitals most of the source population would attend.	No = 0
Internal validity - bias		
14	*Was an attempt made to blind study subjects to the intervention they have received?* For studies where the patients would have no way of knowing which intervention they received, this should be answered yes.[d]	Unable to determine = 0
15	*Was an attempt made to blind those measuring the main outcomes of the intervention?*[d]	Unable to determine = 0
16	*If any of the results of the study were based on "data dredging", was this made clear?* Any analyses that had not been planned at the outset of the study should be clearly indicated. If no retrospective unplanned subgroup analyses were reported, then answer yes.	Unable to determine = 0

Item	Criteria	Answers
17	*In trials and cohort studies, do the analyses adjust for different lengths of follow-up of patients, or in case–control studies, is the time period between the intervention and outcome the same for cases and controls?* Where follow-up was the same for all study patients, the answer should be yes. If different lengths of follow-up were adjusted for by, for example, survival analysis the answer should be yes. Studies where differences in follow-up are ignored should be answered no.	Unable to determine = 0
18	*Were the statistical tests used to assess the main outcomes appropriate?* The statistical techniques used must be appropriate to the data. For example, nonparametric methods should be used for small sample sizes. Where little statistical analysis has been undertaken but where there is no evidence of bias, the question should be answered yes. If the distribution of the data (normal or not) is not described, it must be assumed that the estimates used were appropriate and the question should be answered yes.	Unable to determine = 0
19	*Was compliance with the intervention/s reliable?* Where there was noncompliance with the allocated treatment or where there was contamination of one group, the question should be answered no. For studies where the effect of any misclassification was likely to bias any association to the null, the question should be answered yes.	Unable to determine = 0
20	*Were the main outcome measures used accurate (valid and reliable)?* For studies where the outcome measures are clearly described, the question should be answered yes. For studies which refer to other work or that demonstrates the outcome measures are accurate, the question should be answered as yes.	Unable to determine = 0
Internal validity – confounding (selection bias)		
21	*Were the patients in different intervention groups (trials and cohort studies) or were the cases and controls (case–control studies) recruited from the same population?* For example, patients for all comparison groups should be selected from the same hospital. The question should be answered, unable to determine for cohort and case–control studies where there is no information concerning the source of patients included in the study.[d]	Unable to determine = 0
22	*Were study subjects in different intervention groups (trials and cohort studies) or were the cases and controls (case–control studies) recruited over the same period of time?* For a study which does not specify the time period over which patients were recruited, the question should be answered as unable to determine.[d]	Unable to determine = 0
23	*Were study subjects randomised to intervention groups?* Studies which state that subjects were randomised should be answered yes except where method of randomisation would not ensure random allocation. For example alternate allocation would score no because it is predictable.[d]	Unable to determine = 0
24	*Was the randomised intervention assignment concealed from both patients and health care staff until recruitment was complete and irrevocable?*[d] All non-randomised studies should be answered no. If assignment was concealed from patients but not from staff, it should be answered no.	Unable to determine = 0
25	*Was there adequate adjustment for confounding in the analyses from which the main findings were drawn?* This question should be answered no for trials if: the main conclusions of the study were based on analyses of treatment rather than intention to treat; the distribution of known confounders in the different treatment groups was not described; or the distribution of known confounders differed between the treatment groups but was not taken into account in the analyses. In non-randomised studies, if the effect of the main confounders was not investigated or confounding was demonstrated but no adjustment was made in the final analyses, the question should be answered as no.[d]	Unable to determine = 0

Item	Criteria	Answers
26	*Were losses of patients to follow-up taken into account?* If the numbers of patients lost to follow-up are not reported, the question should be answered as unable to determine. If the proportion lost to follow-up was too small to affect the main findings, the question should be answered yes.	No = 0
Power		
27*	*Was a power analysis performed?*[d]	No = 0

**Modified from the original form published by Downs and Black.*
[a]Sex, age, hypertrophic lesions, Fitzpatrick skin phototype, and previous treatments were considered principal confounders that should be reported in both controlled and uncontrolled studies.
[b]Studies wherein all individual outcome scores have been reported but not variability parameters the item was answered yes (because variability parameters can be derived retrospectively).
[c]Item was answered 'yes' when no statistical tests were performed.
[d]Item numbers 14, 15, and 21–25.

Table C1.
The modified Downs and Black checklist.

Author details

Matome M. Sekhotha*, Pholoso V. Ngwana, Maanda Ravhutendele, Thabang O.L. Sekhotha and Onkgopotse O. Ntsoane
Faculty of Science and Agriculture, School of Molecular Science and Agriculture, Department of Physiology and Environmental Health, University of Limpopo, Sovenga, South Africa

*Address all correspondence to: michael.sekhotha@ul.ac.za

References

[1] López-Pelayo H, Aubin H, Drummond C, Dom G, Pascual F, Rehm J, et al. "The post-COVID era": Challenges in the treatment of substance use disorder (SUD) after the pandemic. BMC Medicine. 2020;**18**:1-8

[2] Tramullas M, Martínez-Cué C, Hurlé MA. Chronic administration of heroin to mice produces up-regulation of brain apoptosis-related proteins and impairs spatial learning and memory. Neuropharmacology. 2008;**54**:640-652. DOI: 10.1016/j.neuropharm.2007.11.018

[3] Bach AG, Jordan B, Wegener NA, Rusner C, Kornhuber M, Abbas J, et al. Heroin spongiform leukoencephalopathy (HSLE). Clinical Neuroradiology. 2012;**22**:345-349. DOI: 10.1007/s00062-012-0173-y

[4] Wang C, Zheng D, Xu J, Lam W, Yew DT. Brain damages in ketamine addicts as revealed by magnetic resonance imaging. Frontiers in Neuroanatomy. 2013;**7**(23):1-8. DOI: 10.3389/fnana.2013.00023

[5] EMCDDA. Trends and Developments. Lisban, Portugal:: European Monitoring Centre for Drugs and Drug Addiction. European Monitoring Centre for Drugs and Drug, Addiction, European Drug Report. 2015

[6] Meyer M, Eichenberger R, Strasser J, Dürsteler KM, Vogel M. «one prick and then it's done»: A mixed-methods exploratory study on intramuscular injection in heroin-assisted treatment. Harm Reduction Journal. 2021;**18**:134. DOI: 10.1186/s12954-021-00584-3

[7] Morton CM, D'Amore N, Nolte K, Bryan P. 'How much heroin is too much heroin?' Youth inquiries regarding opioids. Drugs: Education, Prevention and Policy. 2021;**28**:240-245. DOI: 10.1080/09687637.2020.1804530

[8] Alexander-Savino CV, Mirowski GW, Culton DA. Mucocutaneous manifestations of recreational drug use. American Journal of Clinical Dermatology. 2024;**25**:281-297. DOI: 10.1007/s40257-023-00835-y

[9] Baldo BA. Toxicities of opioid analgesics: Respiratory depression, histamine release, hemodynamic changes, hypersensitivity, serotonin toxicity. Archives of Toxicology. 2021;**95**:2627-2642. DOI: 10.1007/s00204-021-03068-2

[10] Elfers K, Menne L, Colnaghi L, Hoppe S, Mazzuoli-Weber G. Short- and long-term effects of cocaine on enteric neuronal functions. Cells. 2023;**12**:577. DOI: 10.3390/cells12040577

[11] Daniels W, Sekhotha M, Morgan N, Manilall A. The cytotoxic effects of Nyaope, a heroin-based street drug, in SH-SY5Y Neuroblastoma cells. IBRO Neuroscience Reports. 2024;**16**:280-290. DOI: 10.1016/j.ibneur.2024.01.014

[12] White CM, Browne T, Nafziger AN. Inherent dangers of using non–US Food and Drug Administration–approved substances of abuse. Journal of Clinical Pharmacology. 2021;**61**(S2):S129-S141. DOI: 10.1002/jcph.1860

[13] Kaleem M, Khan S. Unveiling the complexities of cocaine. Forensic Insights and Health Sciences Bulletin. 2024;**2**:1-10. Available from: https://ammanif.com/journal/fi/index.php/home/article/view/139

[14] Khine A, Mokwena K, Huma M, Fernandes L. Identifying the composition

of street drug Nyaope using two different mass spectrometer methods. African Journal of Drug & Alcohol Studies. 2015;**14**:49-56

[15] Mthembi PM, Mwenesongole EM, Cole MD. Chemical profiling of the street cocktail drug 'nyaope' in South Africa using GC–MS II: Stability studies of the cannabinoid, opiate and antiretroviral components during sample storage. Forensic Science International. 2019;**300**:187-192. DOI: 10.1016/j.forsciint.2019.04.040

[16] Schneider S, Richter C, Niethammer R, Beisel L. Fatal and non-fatal heroin-related overdoses: Circumstances and patterns. Substance Use & Misuse. 2021;**56**:1997-2006. DOI: 10.1080/10826084.2021.1963986

[17] Choi JI, Lee J, Yeh AB, Lan Q, Kang H. Spatial clustering of heroin-related overdose incidents: A case study in Cincinnati, Ohio. BMC Public Health. 2022;**22**:1253. DOI: 10.1186/s12889-022-13557-3

[18] McNair R, Monaghan M, Montgomery P. Heroin assisted treatment for key health outcomes in people with chronic heroin addictions: A context-focused systematic review. Drug and Alcohol Dependence. 2023;**247**:109869. DOI: 10.1016/j.drugalcdep.2023.109869

[19] Caglioni M, Ragona A, Maremmani A, Silvia C, Cerniglia L. The impact of COVID-19 pandemic on pregnant women with substance use disorder: A narrative review. Heroin Addiction And Related Clinical Problems. 2022;**24**:1-9. Available from: https://www.heroinaddictionrelatedclinicalproblems.org/harcp-archives-doi-articles.php

[20] Boyd S. Heroin and the illegal drug overdose death epidemic: A history of missed opportunities and resistance. The International Journal on Drug Policy. 2021;**91**:102938. DOI: 10.1016/j.drugpo.2020.102938

[21] Gutierrez A, Harvey EL, Creehan KM, Taffe MA. The long-term effects of repeated heroin vapor inhalation during adolescence on measures of nociception and anxiety-like behavior in adult Wistar rats. Psychopharmacology. 2022;**239**:3939-3952. DOI: 10.1007/s00213-022-06267-6

[22] Yue Y, Zou L, Li H, Xia Y, Ren Z, Yang F, et al. Therapeutic effect of implanted and non-invasive vagus nerve stimulation on heroin-induced anxiety. Biochemical and Biophysical Research Communications. 2023;**652**:46-54. DOI: 10.1016/j.bbrc.2023.02.041

[23] Mirković-Hajdukov M, Efendić-Spahić T, Šakušić A, Bećirović E, Softić R, Kunić S. Emotional profile of heroine addicts. Acta Medica Saliniana. 2021;**51**:36-40. DOI: 10.5457/ams.v51i1-2.581

[24] Jacobson M, Browne C, Lucki I. Kappa opioid receptor antagonists as potential therapeutics for stress-related disorders. Annual Review of Pharmacology and Toxicology. 2020;**60**:615-636

[25] Dowell D, Ragan K, Jones C, Baldwin G, Chou R. Prescribing opioids for pain—The new CDC clinical practice guideline. The New England Journal of Medicine. 2022;**387**:2011-2013

[26] Marel C, Wilson J, Darke S, Ross J, Slade T, Haber PS, et al. Patterns and predictors of heroin use, remission, and psychiatric health among people with heroin dependence: Key findings from the 18-20-year follow-up of the Australian treatment outcome study (ATOS). International Journal of Mental

Health & Addiction. 2024;**22**:2565-2582. DOI: 10.1007/s11469-022-01006-6

[27] Maremmani I, Pacini M, Maremmani AGI. Chronic psychosis in dual disorder heroin use disorder patients. In: Dual Disord. Heroin Addicts. Cham: Springer Nature Switzerland; 2023. pp. 109-163. DOI: 10.1007/978-3-031-30093-6_4

[28] Tolomeo S, Steele JD, Ekhtiari H, Baldacchino A. Chronic heroin use disorder and the brain: Current evidence and future implications. Progress in Neuro-Psychopharmacology & Biological Psychiatry. 2021;**111**:110148. DOI: 10.1016/j.pnpbp.2020.110148

[29] Mas-Herrero E, Ferreri L, Cardona G, Zatorre R, Pla-Juncà F, Antonijoan R, et al. The role of opioid transmission in music-induced pleasure. Annals of the New York Academy of Sciences. 2023;**1520**:105-114

[30] Rogers A, Garey L, Bakhshaie J, Viana A, Ditre J, Zvolensky M. Anxiety, depression, and opioid misuse among adults with chronic pain: The role of anxiety sensitivity. The Clinical Journal of Pain. 2020;**36**:862-867

[31] Friedman S, Krawczyk N, Perlman D, Mateu-Gelabert P, Ompad D, Hamilton L, et al. The opioid/overdose crisis as a dialectics of pain, despair, and one-sided struggle. Frontiers in Public Health. 2020;**8**:540423

[32] Bateman J, Saunders S, Levitt E. Understanding and countering opioid-induced respiratory depression. British Journal of Pharmacology. 2023;**180**:813-828

[33] Cutrufello N, Ianus V, Rowley J. Opioids and sleep. Current Opinion in Pulmonary Medicine. 2020;**26**:634-641

[34] Valbrun L, Zvonarev V. The opioid system and food intake: Use of opiate antagonists in treatment of binge eating disorder and abnormal eating behavior. Journal of Clinical Medical Research. 2020;**12**:41

[35] Viscusi E, Viscusi A. Blood–brain barrier: Mechanisms governing permeability and interaction with peripherally acting μ-opioid receptor antagonists. Regional Anesthesia and Pain Medicine. 2020;**45**:688-695. DOI: 10.1136/rapm-2020-101403

[36] Reeves K, Shah N, Muñoz B, Atwood B. Opioid receptor-mediated regulation of neurotransmission in the brain. Frontiers in Molecular Neuroscience. 2022;**15**:e919773. DOI: 10.3389/fnmol.2022.919773

[37] Jaschke N, Pählig S, Pan Y, Hofbauer L, Göbel A, Rachner T. From pharmacology to physiology: Endocrine functions of μ-opioid receptor networks. Trends in Endocrinology and Metabolism. 2021;**32**:306-319

[38] Wu D, Chen Q, Chen X, Han F, Chen Z, Wang Y. The blood–brain barrier: Structure, regulation and drug delivery. Signal Transduction and Targeted Therapy. 2023;**8**:217. DOI: 10.1038/s41392-023-01481-w

[39] Sescil J, Havens SM, Wang W. Principles and design of molecular tools for sensing and perturbing cell surface receptor activity. Chemical Reviews. 2025;**15**:e919773, pp. 2665-2702. DOI: 10.1021/acs.chemrev.4c00582

[40] Massaccesi C, Korb S, Willeit M, Quednow B, Silani G. Effects of the mu-opioid receptor agonist morphine on facial mimicry and emotion recognition. Psychoneuroendocrinology. 2022;**142**:105801

[41] Moustafa A, Tindle R, Cashel S, Parkes D, Mohamed E, Abo Hamza E. Bidirectional relationship between heroin addiction and depression: Behavioural and neural studies. Current Psychology. 2020;**41**(8):5195-5211

[42] Milella M, D'Ottavio G, De Pirro S, Barra M, Caprioli D, Badiani A. Heroin and its metabolites: Relevance to heroin use disorder. Translational Psychiatry. 2023;**13**:120

[43] Sideli L, Quigley H, La Cascia C, Murray R. Cannabis use and the risk for psychosis and affective disorders. Journal of Dual Diagnosis. 2020;**16**:22-42

[44] Mella-Raipán J, Romero-Parra J, Recabarren-Gajardo G. DARK classics in chemical neuroscience: Heroin and desomorphine. ACS Chemical Neuroscience. 2020;**11**:3905-3927

[45] Kerrigan S, Goldberger BA. Opioids. In: Levine BS, Kerrigan S, editors. Principles of Forensic Toxicology. Cham: Springer; 2020. DOI: 10.1007/978-3-030-42917-1_22

[46] Vearrier D, Grundmann O. Clinical pharmacology, toxicity, and abuse potential of opioids. Journal of Clinical Pharmacology. 2021;**61**(S2):S70-S88. DOI: 10.1002/jcph.1923

[47] George BE, Dawes MH, Peck EG, Jones SR. Altered accumbal dopamine terminal dynamics following chronic heroin self-administration. International Journal of Molecular Sciences. 2022;**23**:8106. DOI: 10.3390/ijms23158106

[48] Megerian CE, Bair L, Smith J, Browne EN, Wenger LD, Guzman L, et al. Health risks associated with smoking versus injecting fentanyl among people who use drugs in California. Drug and Alcohol Dependence. 2024;**255**:111053. DOI: 10.1016/j.drugalcdep.2023.111053

[49] Strang J. Heroin and cocaine: New technologies, new problems. In: Addiction Controversies. London: CRC Press; 2023. pp. 201-211

[50] Qiu Y, Wang Y-J. Editorial: Opioids and opioid receptors in pain, addiction, and mood disorders. Frontiers in Psychiatry. 2024;**15**:711-723. DOI: 10.3389/fpsyt.2024.1382894

[51] Kong Y. Mechanisms of opioids and evaluation on existing therapies for addiction. MATEC Web of Conferences. 2024;**404**:04002. DOI: 10.1051/matecconf/202440404002

[52] Cruz SL, Paz-Ramos MI, Hernández-Mendoza A, Carranza-Aguilar CJ. Opioid Effects and Classification. Opioids, Cham: Springer International Publishing; 2022. pp. 149-174. DOI: 10.1007/978-3-031-09936-6_8

[53] Kesten JM, Holder E, Ayres R, Ellis P, Taylor S, Hickman M, et al. Changes in the development of opioid tolerance on re-exposure among people who use heroin: A qualitative study. PLoS One. 2022;**17**:e0269379. DOI: 10.1371/journal.pone.0269379

[54] Gipson CD, Dunn KE, Bull A, Ulangkaya H, Hossain A. Establishing preclinical withdrawal syndrome symptomatology following heroin self-administration in male and female rats. Experimental and Clinical Psychopharmacology. 2021;**29**:636-649. DOI: 10.1037/pha0000375

[55] Wang S, Zhang M, Liu S, Xu Y, Shao Z, Chen L, et al. Impulsivity in heroin-dependent individuals: Structural and functional abnormalities within frontostriatal circuits. Brain Imaging and Behavior.

2021;**15**:2454-2463. DOI: 10.1007/s11682-020-00445-w

[56] Xu W, Hong Q, Lin Z, Ma H, Chen W, Zhuang D, et al. Role of nucleus accumbens microRNA-181a and MeCP2 in incubation of heroin craving in male rats. Psychopharmacology. 2021;**238**:2313-2324. DOI: 10.1007/s00213-021-05854-3

[57] Feng Y, He X, Yang Y, Chao DH, Lazarus L, Xia Y. Current research on opioid receptor function. Current Drug Targets. 2012;**13**:230-246. DOI: 10.2174/138945012799201612

[58] Morgan J, Bennett T. The nature and implications of lifestyle transitions for persistent heroin use. Contemporary Drug Problems. 2023;**50**:541-555. DOI: 10.1177/00914509231189934

[59] Su H, Yang L, Cao H, Zhang J, Li X, Li Y. Effect of automatic emotional processing on response inhibition among heroin abstainers. PsyCh Journal. 2022;**11**:913-921. DOI: 10.1002/pchj.574

[60] Brooks SK, Webster RK, Smith LE, Woodland L, Wessely S, Greenberg N, et al. The psychological impact of quarantine and how to reduce it: Rapid review of the evidence. Lancet. 2020;**395**:912-920. DOI: 10.1016/S0140-6736(20)30460-8

[61] Salmanzadeh H, Ahmadi-Soleimani S, Pachenari N, Azadi M, Halliwell R, Rubino T, et al. Adolescent drug exposure: A review of evidence for the development of persistent changes in brain function. Brain Research Bulletin. 2020;**156**:105-117

[62] Luo Y, Liao C, Chen L, Zhang Y, Bao S, Deng A, et al. Heroin addiction induces axonal transport dysfunction in the brain detected by In vivo MRI. Neurotoxicity Research. 2022;**40**:1070-1085. DOI: 10.1007/s12640-022-00533-3

[63] Müller UJ, Ahrens M, Vasilevska V, Dobrowolny H, Schiltz K, Schlaaff K, et al. Reduced habenular volumes and neuron numbers in male heroin addicts: A post-mortem study. European Archives of Psychiatry and Clinical Neuroscience. 2021;**271**:835-845. DOI: 10.1007/s00406-020-01195-y

[64] Abboud C, Duveau A, Bouali-Benazzouz R, Massé K, Mattar J, Brochoire L, et al. Animal models of pain: Diversity and benefits. Journal of Neuroscience Methods. 2021;**348**:108997

[65] Gong X, Cheng D, Li W, Shen Y, Peng R, Shi L, et al. A highly selective ratiometric molecular probe for imaging peroxynitrite during drug-induced acute liver injury. Journal of Materials Chemistry B. 2021;**9**:8246-8252

[66] Raza M, Su S. Differential roles for dopamine D1-like and D2-like receptors in learning and behavior of honeybee and other insects. Applied Ecology and Environmental Research. 2020;**18**:1317-1327. Aviable from: https://aloki.hu/pdf/1801_13171327.pdf

[67] Winstanley EL, Mahoney JJ, Castillo F, Comer SD. Neurocognitive impairments and brain abnormalities resulting from opioid-related overdoses: A systematic review. Drug and Alcohol Dependence. 2021;**226**:108838. DOI: 10.1016/j.drugalcdep.2021.108838

[68] Sekhotha MM, Sekhotha TOL. The effect of administration of substance abuse among people suffering from substance use disorder on the digestive system: A systematic review. In: Monyeki KD, Kemper HCG, Modjadji P, editors. Metabolic Syndrome - Lifestyle and Biological Risk Factors. Rijeka:

IntechOpen; 2024. DOI: 10.5772/intechopen.115034

[69] Sekhotha M, Daniels W, Muller D, Malatswana S, Mathikhi K, Mokwena T, et al. Nyaope consumption by south African youth-reflections on the neglect of rehabilitation centres for substance use disorder: A systematic review. African Journal for Physical Activity and Health Sciences. 2023;**29**:89-117

[70] Weiten W. The biological bases of behavior. Psychology, Thomson; 2006, p. 73-98

[71] Azimi S, Docoslis A. Recent advances in the use of surface-enhanced Raman scattering for illicit drug detection. Sensors. 2022;**22**:3877. DOI: 10.3390/s22103877

[72] Paz-Ramos MI, Cruz SL, Violante-Soria V. Amphetamine-type stimulants: Novel insights into their actions and use patterns. Revista de Investigación Clínica. 2023;**75**(3):143-157. DOI: 10.24875/RIC.23000110

[73] Dresp-Langley B. From reward to anhedonia-dopamine function in the global mental health context. Biomedicine. 2023;**11**:2469. DOI: 10.3390/biomedicines11092469

[74] Martins F, NHC L, el Yattouti M, Offeringa L, Heydari P, MJX H, et al. P-glycoprotein (MDR1/ABCB1) restricts brain penetration of the Main active heroin metabolites 6-monoacetylmorphine (6-MAM) and morphine in mice. Pharmaceutical Research. 2023;**40**:1885-1899. DOI: 10.1007/s11095-023-03545-6

[75] Marie N, Noble F. Oxycodone, an opioid like the others? Front. Psychiatry. 2023;**14**:e1229439. DOI: 10.3389/fpsyt.2023.1229439

[76] Cameron-Burr KT, Conicella A, Neavyn MJ. Opioid use and driving performance. Journal of Medical Toxicology. 2021;**17**:289-308. DOI: 10.1007/s13181-020-00819-y

[77] Di Chiara G, Imperato A. Drugs abused by humans preferentially increase synaptic dopamine concentrations in the mesolimbic system of freely moving rats. Proceedings of the National Academy of Sciences. 1988;**85**:5274-5278. DOI: 10.1073/pnas.85.14.5274

[78] Martinez S, Brandt L, Comer SD, Levin FR, Jones JD. The subjective experience of heroin effects among individuals with chronic opioid use: Revisiting reinforcement in an exploratory study. Addiction Neuroscience. 2022;**4**:100034. DOI: 10.1016/j.addicn.2022.100034

[79] Duhart Clarke SE, Kral AH, Zibbell JE. Consuming illicit opioids during a drug overdose epidemic: Illicit fentanyls, drug discernment, and the radical transformation of the illicit opioid market. The International Journal on Drug Policy. 2022;**99**:103467. DOI: 10.1016/j.drugpo.2021.103467

[80] Igwe CN, Robinson F, Jones SM. A novel case of ocular cicatricial pemphigoid induced by levamisole-adulterated cocaine. European Journal of Ophthalmology. 2021;**31**:11-15. DOI: 10.1177/1120672120964756

[81] Costello BJ, Anderson BJ, Stein M. Peer influence in initiation to heroin use. Journal of Drug Issues. 2021;**51**:323-339. DOI: 10.1177/0022042620979628

[82] Calcaterra SL, Lockhart S, Callister C, Hoover K, Binswanger IA. Opioid use disorder treatment initiation and continuation: A qualitative study

of patients who received addiction consultation and hospital-based providers. Journal of General Internal Medicine. 2022;**37**:2786-2794. DOI: 10.1007/s11606-021-07305-3

[83] Breiter H, Gollub R, Weisskoff R, Kennedy D, Makris N, Berke J, et al. Acute effects of cocaine on human brain activity and emotion. Neuron. 1997;**19**:591-611

[84] Patel A, Poddar S, Nierenberg D, Lang S, Wang H, Pires DeMello CP, et al. Microphysiological system to address the opioid crisis: A novel multi-organ model of acute opioid overdose and recovery. Current Research in Toxicology. 2025;**8**:100209. DOI: 10.1016/j.crtox.2024.100209

[85] Roque Bravo R, Faria AC, Brito-da-Costa AM, Carmo H, Mladěnka P, Dias da Silva D, et al. Cocaine: An updated overview on chemistry, detection, biokinetics, and pharmacotoxicological aspects including abuse pattern. Toxins (Basel). 2022;**14**:278. DOI: 10.3390/toxins14040278

[86] Della Rocca F, Maremmani AGI, Bacciardi S, Pacini M, Lamanna F, Tripodi B, et al. Characteristics of stress sensitivity in heroin use disorder patients during their opioid agonist treatment. International Journal of Environmental Research and Public Health. 2023;**20**:4566. DOI: 10.3390/ijerph20054566

[87] Varadarajan V, Ibe CA, Young JH. Effect of substance use on premature mortality among severely hypertensive African Americans. Journal of Clinical Hypertension. 2022;**24**:475-482. DOI: 10.1111/jch.14420

[88] Keogh CF, Andrews GT, Spacey SD, Forkheim KE, Graeb DA. Neuroimaging features of heroin inhalation toxicity: "Chasing the dragon". American Journal of Roentgenology. 2003;**180**:847-850. DOI: 10.2214/ajr.180.3.1800847

[89] Sharifian-Dorche M, La Piana R. General approach to treatment of genetic leukoencephalopathies in children and adults. 2024;**204**:335-354. DOI: 10.1016/B978-0-323-99209-1.00012-0

[90] Diefenbach C, Lorenz C, Weidauer S. Toxic spongiform leukoencephalopathy after intravenous heroin abuse: Unusual but important differential diagnosis of acute impairment of consciousness. Fortschritte der Neurologie, Psychiatrie. 2022;**90**:523-528. DOI: 10.1055/a-1778-3662

[91] Vasconcelos LP, Gandini JG, Teixeir AL, Manto M. Movement disorders associated with stimulants and other drugs of abuse. In: Teixeira A, Stimming EF, Ondo WG, editors. Movement Disorders in Psychiatry. online edn. New York: Oxford Academic; 1 Sept 2022. DOI: 10.1093/ med/9780197574317.003.0009 [Accessed 2 Apr. 2025]

[92] Yildirim E, Selcuk M, Saylik F, Mutluer FO, Deniz O. Efeitos da Heroína nos Parâmetros Eletrocardiográficos. Arquivos Brasileiros de Cardiologia. 2020;**115**:1135-1411. DOI: 10.36660/abc.20190296

[93] Thomas SA, Curay CM, Kiyatkin EA. Relationships between oxygen changes in the brain and periphery following physiological activation and the actions of heroin and cocaine. Scientific Reports. 2021;**11**:6355. DOI: 10.1038/s41598-021-85798-y

[94] Gaudreault P-O, King SG, Malaker P, Alia-Klein N, Goldstein RZ. Whole-brain white matter abnormalities in human cocaine and heroin use disorders:

Association with craving, recency, and cumulative use. Molecular Psychiatry. 2023;**28**:780-791. DOI: 10.1038/s41380-022-01833-y

[95] Zhu J, Yan X, Lyu Z, Wang S, Chen J, Wang W, et al. Characteristics of white matter integrity during different phases of abstinence in heroin use disorders: A diffusion tensor imaging study. Journal of Addiction Medicine. 2022;**16**:541-548. DOI: 10.1097/ADM.0000000000000962

[96] Alshamam MS, Sumbly V, Nso N, Saliaj M, Gurung DO. Heroin-Induced Leukoencephalopathy. Cureus. 2021:e13093. DOI: 10.7759/cureus.13093

[97] Farrell A, O'Brien B, Janeczko P, Cassimatis N, Monoky D. Heroin inhalation leukoencephalopathy: An overlooked entity in the opioid epidemic. Cureus. 2023:e40535. DOI: 10.7759/cureus.40535

[98] Hassan WA, Shehata S, ElBana A. Histopathological Assessment of the Effect of Pregabalin Toxicity on Cerebrum and Cerebellum of Adult Albino Rats2021. DOI: 10.21203/rs.3.rs-149289/v1

[99] Mitaritonno M, Lupo M, Greco I, Mazza A, Cervellin G. Severe rhabdomyolysis induced by co-administration of cocaine and heroin in a 45 years old man treated with rosuvastatin: A case report. Acta Biomed. 2021;**92**(S1):e2021089. DOI: 10.23750/abm.v92iS1.8858

[100] Griffin K, Stitt D. Opioid-associated nervous system injuries. Seminars in Neurology. 2024;**44**:452-458. DOI: 10.1055/s-0044-1787545

[101] Kiyatkin EA. Hypoxic effects of heroin and fentanyl and their basic physiological mechanisms. American Journal of Physiology-Cell Physiology. 2024;**327**:L930-L948. DOI: 10.1152/ajplung.00251.2024

[102] Fadhil F. Post-Traumatic Risk Factors in Heroin Addiction Patients Undergoing Substitution Treatment. International Journal of Social Science and Humanity. 2021;**20**. DOI: 10.33193/IJoHSS.20.2021.233

[103] Carr CM, Benson JC, DeLone DR, Diehn FE, Kim DK, Merrell KW, et al. Intracranial long-term complications of radiation therapy: An image-based review. Neuroradiology. 2021;**63**:471-482. DOI: 10.1007/s00234-020-02621-7

[104] Nuqui PBE, Hernandez FG. Chemotherapy-induced leukoencephalopathy: A case series. Journal of Medicine, University of Santo Tomas. 2021;**5**:658-663. DOI: 10.35460/2546-1621.2019-0057

[105] Nigro SE, Hall LP, Harman J, Willard VW, Conklin HM, Pui C-H, et al. The association of environmental factors with neurocognitive outcomes in survivors of childhood acute lymphoblastic leukemia (ALL). Support Care Cancer. 2024;**32**:1. DOI: 10.1007/s00520-023-08212-5

[106] Bajwa MS, Nawaz H, Ur Rehman MA, Iftikhar S, Hurera A. Leukoencephalopathy due to inhalational and trans-conjunctival heroin abuse: First case report from Pakistan. Annals of Medicine and Surgery. 2022;**75**. DOI: 10.1016/j.amsu.2022.103351

[107] Agarwal A, Rees JH, Sabat S. Toxic and drug-related white matter diseases of the brain and spine. Magnetic Resonance Imaging Clinics of North America. 2024;**32**:253-275. DOI: 10.1016/j.mric.2023.12.002

[108] Knudsen GH, Kermanian N, Kock-Jensen CH, Antulov R.

Opioid-induced leukoencephalopathies: A report of two cases. Case Reports in Neurology. 2022;**14**:25-30. DOI: 10.1159/000521410

[109] Ahmed U, Wilson R, Hung S-C. Bilateral cerebellar hemorrhagic infarcts as an early presentation following opioid-induced toxic encephalopathy in an adult patient. Radiology Case Reports. 2021;**16**:1207-1210. DOI: 10.1016/j.radcr.2021.02.073

[110] Hoogeveen ES, Pelzer N, Ghariq E, van Osch MJ, Dahan A, Terwindt GM, et al. Cerebrovascular reactivity in retinal vasculopathy with cerebral leukoencephalopathy and systemic manifestations. Journal of Cerebral Blood Flow and Metabolism. 2021;**41**:831-840. DOI: 10.1177/0271678X20929430

[111] Argirò A, Sciagrà R, Marchi A, Beltrami M, Spinelli E, Salvadori E, et al. Coronary microvascular function is impaired in patients with cerebral autosomal dominant arteriopathy with subcortical infarcts and leukoencephalopathy. European Journal of Neurology. 2021;**28**:3809-3813. DOI: 10.1111/ene.14678

[112] Bennett CF, Latorre-Muro P, Puigserver P. Mechanisms of mitochondrial respiratory adaptation. Nature Reviews. Molecular Cell Biology. 2022;**23**:817-835. DOI: 10.1038/s41580-022-00506-6

[113] McGrath SP, McGovern KM, Perreard IM, Huang V, Moss LB, Blike GT. Inpatient respiratory arrest associated with sedative and analgesic medications: Impact of continuous monitoring on patient mortality and severe morbidity. Journal of Patient Safety. 2021;**17**:557-561. DOI: 10.1097/PTS.0000000000000696

[114] Haouzi P, Tubbs N. Effects of fentanyl overdose-induced muscle rigidity and dexmedetomidine on respiratory mechanics and pulmonary gas exchange in sedated rats. Journal of Applied Physiology. 2022;**132**:1407-1422. DOI: 10.1152/japplphysiol.00819.2021

[115] Kiyatkin E, Choi S. Brain oxygen responses induced by opioids: Focus on heroin, fentanyl, and their adulterants. Frontiers in Psychiatry. 2024;**15**:1354722

[116] Fonseca NM, Guimarães GMN, Pontes JPJ, Ávila Oliveira R. Safety and effectiveness of adding fentanyl or sufentanil to spinal anesthesia: Systematic review and meta-analysis of randomized controlled trials. Brazilian Journal of Anesthesiology (English Edition). 2023;**73**:198-216. DOI: 10.1016/j.bjane.2021.10.010

[117] Patocka J, Wu W, Oleksak P, Jelinkova R, Nepovimova E, Spicanova L, et al. Fentanyl and its derivatives: Pain-killers or man-killers? Heliyon. 2024;**10**:e28795. DOI: 10.1016/j.heliyon.2024.e28795

[118] Zellner T, Eyer F, Rabe C, Geith S, Haberl B, Schmoll S. Recreational drug overdose—Clinical value of toxicological analysis. Toxics. 2024;**12**:662. DOI: 10.3390/toxics12090662

[119] Friedman J, Godvin M, Molina C, Romero R, Borquez A, Avra T, et al. Fentanyl, heroin, and methamphetamine-based counterfeit pills sold at tourist-oriented pharmacies in Mexico: An ethnographic and drug checking study. Drug and Alcohol Dependence. 2023;**249**:110819. DOI: 10.1016/j.drugalcdep.2023.110819

[120] Kariisa M, O'Donnell J, Kumar S, Mattson CL, Goldberger BA. Illicitly Manufactured Fentanyl–Involved Overdose Deaths with Detected

Xylazine—United States, January 2019–June 2022. MMWR. Morbidity and Mortality Weekly Report. 2023;**72**:721-727. DOI: 10.15585/mmwr.mm7226a4

[121] Jeffery MM, Stevens M, D'Onofrio G, Melnick ER. Fentanyl-associated overdose deaths outside the hospital. The New England Journal of Medicine. 2023;**389**:87-88. DOI: 10.1056/NEJMc2304991

[122] Moss LM, Algera MH, Dobbins R, Gray F, Strafford S, Heath A, et al. Effect of sustained high buprenorphine plasma concentrations on fentanyl-induced respiratory depression: A placebo-controlled crossover study in healthy volunteers and opioid-tolerant patients. PLoS One. 2022;**17**:e0256752. DOI: 10.1371/journal.pone.0256752

[123] Olofsen E, Algera MH, Moss L, Dobbins RL, Groeneveld GJ, van Velzen M, et al. Modeling buprenorphine reduction of fentanyl-induced respiratory depression. JCI Insight. 2022;7(9):e156973. DOI: 10.1172/jci.insight.156973

[124] Pyar K, Hlaing S, Aung A, Aung Z, Hla S, Aung S, et al. Fentanyl overdose presented with unconsciousness, hypoxia, hypotension and pinpoint pupil complicated by acute kidney injury and right hemiparesis: A rare case report. Clin. Cardiovascular Research. 2023;**2**. DOI: 10.58489/2836-5917/009

[125] Pietsch U, Fischer H, Rüst CA, Hossfeld B, Grünenfelder A, Wenzel V, et al. Oral transmucosal fentanyl citrate analgesia in prehospital trauma care: An observational cohort study. Scandinavian Journal of Trauma, Resuscitation and Emergency Medicine. 2023;**31**:2. DOI: 10.1186/s13049-023-01066-0

[126] Getsy PM, Baby SM, May WJ, Lewis THJ, Bates JN, Hsieh Y-H, et al. L-NAC reverses of the adverse effects of fentanyl infusion on ventilation and blood-gas chemistry. Biomedicine & Pharmacotherapy. 2022;**153**:113277. DOI: 10.1016/j.biopha.2022.113277

[127] Bates JN, Baby SM, Getsy PM, Coffee GA, Hsieh Y-H, Knauss ZT, et al. L-NAC and L-NAC methyl ester prevent and overcome physical dependence to fentanyl in male rats. Scientific Reports. 2024;**14**:9091. DOI: 10.1038/s41598-024-59551-0

[128] Quintanilla ME, Morales P, Santapau D, Gallardo J, Rebolledo R, Riveras G, et al. Morphine self-administration is inhibited by the antioxidant N-acetylcysteine and the anti-inflammatory ibudilast; an effect enhanced by their co-administration. PLoS One. 2024;**19**:e0312828. DOI: 10.1371/journal.pone.0312828

[129] Downs AM, Kmiec G, McElligott ZA. Oral fentanyl consumption and withdrawal impairs fear extinction learning and enhances basolateral amygdala principal neuron excitatory-inhibitory balance in male and female mice. Addiction Neuroscience. 2024;**13**:100182. DOI: 10.1016/j.addicn.2024.100182

[130] Choi S, Noya MR, Kiyatkin EA. Oxygen fluctuations in the brain and periphery induced by intravenous fentanyl: Effects of dose and drug experience. Journal of Neurophysiology. 2024;**132**:322-334. DOI: 10.1152/jn.00177.2024

[131] Koekkoek LL, van der Gun LL, Serlie MJ, la Fleur SE. The clash of two epidemics: The relationship between opioids and glucose metabolism. Current Diabetes Reports. 2022;**22**:301-310. DOI: 10.1007/s11892-022-01473-0

[132] Kiyatkin E. Respiratory depression and brain hypoxia induced by opioid

drugs: Morphine, oxycodone, heroin, and fentanyl. Neuropharmacology. 2019;**151**:219-226

[133] Onaolapo O, Olofinnade A, Ojo F, Adeleye O, Falade J, Onaolapo A. Substance use and substance use disorders in Africa: An epidemiological approach to the review of existing literature. World Psychiatry Journal. 2022;**12**:1268-1286. DOI: 10.5498/wjp.v12.i10.1268

[134] Huỳnh C, Kisely S, Rochette L, Pelletier É, Jutras-Aswad D, Larocque A, et al. Using administrative health data to estimate prevalence and mortality rates of alcohol and other substance-related disorders for surveillance purposes. Drug and Alcohol Review. 2021;**40**:662-672. DOI: 10.1111/dar.13235

[135] Gentile A, Bianco A, Nordström A, Nordström P. Use of alcohol, drugs, inhalants, and smoking tobacco and the long-term risk of depression in men: A nationwide Swedish cohort study from 1969-2017. Drug and Alcohol Dependence. 2021;**221**:108553. DOI: 10.1016/j.drugalcdep.2021.108553

[136] Madiga M, Mokwena K. Depression symptoms among family members of Nyaope users in the City of Tshwane, South Africa. International Journal of Environmental Research and Public Health. 2022;**19**:4097. DOI: 10.3390/ijerph19074097

[137] Morgan N, Daniels W, Subramaney U. A prospective observational study of heroin users in Johannesburg, South Africa: Assessing psychiatric comorbidities and treatment outcomes. Comprehensive Psychiatry. 2019;**95**:152137. DOI: 10.1016/j.comppsych.2019.152137

[138] Semaan A, Khan MK. Neurobiology of Addiction. 2025. Available from: https://pubmed.ncbi.nlm.nih.gov/37983351/

[139] Turski WA, Cavalheiro EA, Ikonomidou C, Mello LE, Bortolotto ZA, Turski L. Effects of aminophylline and 2-chloroadenosine on seizures produced by pilocarpine in rats: Morphological and electroencephalographic correlates. Brain Research. 1985;**361**:309-323. DOI: 10.1016/0006-8993(85)91302-2

[140] Meyer JS, Brevard ME, Piper BJ, Ali SF, Ferris CF. Neural effects of MDMA as determined by functional magnetic resonance imaging and magnetic resonance spectroscopy in awake marmoset monkeys. Annals of the New York Academy of Sciences. 2006;**1074**:365-376. DOI: 10.1196/annals.1369.036

[141] Offiah C, Hall E. Heroin-induced leukoencephalopathy: Characterization using MRI, diffusion-weighted imaging, and MR spectroscopy. Clinical Radiology. 2008;**63**:146-152

[142] Wang X, Li B, Zhou X, Liao Y, Tang J, Liu T, et al. Changes in brain gray matter in abstinent heroin addicts. Drug and Alcohol Dependence. 2012;**126**:304-308

[143] Solis E, Cameron-Burr K, Shaham Y, Kiyatkin E. Fentanyl-induced brain hypoxia triggers brain hyperglycemia and biphasic changes in brain temperature. Neuropsychopharmacology. 2018;**43**:810-819

[144] Kashyap S, Majeed G, Bowen I, Beamer Y, Miulli D. Toxic leukoencephalopathy due to inhalational heroin abuse. Annals of Indian Academy of Neurology. 2020;**23**:542-544

[145] Bosco F, Guarnieri L, Leo A, Tallarico M, Gallelli L, Rania V, et al.

Audiogenic epileptic DBA/2 mice strain as a model of genetic reflex seizures and SUDEP. Frontiers in Neurology. 2023;**14**:1223074

[146] Boitor M, Ballard A, Emed J, Le May S, Gélinas C. Risk factors for severe opioid-induced respiratory depression in hospitalized adults: A case–control study. Can. The Journal of Pain. 2020;**4**(1):103-110. DOI: 10.1080/24740527.2020.1714431

[147] Saadatnia M, Norouzi R, Najafi MA, Gol Parvar S, Najafian A, Tabatabei A, et al. Opioid use disorder and intracerebral hemorrhage in Isfahan, Iran: A case–control study. Frontiers in Neurology. 2024;**15**:e1420675. DOI: 10.3389/fneur.2024.1420675

[148] Kar H, Gania A, Bandy A, Ud Din Dar N, Rafiq F. Psychiatric comorbidities and concurrent substance use among people who inject drugs: A single-Centre hospital-based study. Scientific Reports. 2023;**13**:19053

[149] Abdelghani M, Fouad AA, Mamdouh A, Raya YM. Association between cognitive impairment and substance use disorder attributed to Pregabalin in Egypt: A case-control study. Addictive Disorders & Their Treatment. 2020;**19**:201-208. DOI: 10.1097/ADT.0000000000000223

[150] Dayyani M, Zabihyan S, Salehi M, Baharvahdat H, Ahmadi S, Etemadrezaie H. Association of opium addiction with rupture of intracranial aneurysms: A case-control study. World Neurosurgery. 2019;**126**:e492-e499. DOI: 10.1016/j.wneu.2019.02.077

[151] Hamziee-Moghadam A, Iranmanesh F, Arabpour-Fathabadi A, Mohammadi F. Cerebrovascular Reactivity and Carotid Intima-Media Thickness in Opium Dependents: A Case-Control Study. Vol. 10. Addict Heal; 2018. pp. 131-136. DOI: 10.22122/ahj.v10i2.555

[152] Barber PA, Pridmore HM, Krishnamurthy V, Roberts S, Spriggs DA, Carter KN, et al. Cannabis, ischemic stroke, and transient ischemic attack. Stroke. 2013;**44**:2327-2329. DOI: 10.1161/STROKEAHA.113.001562

[153] Walker JM, Farney RJ, Rhondeau SM, Boyle KM, Valentine K, Cloward TV, et al. Chronic opioid use is a risk factor for the development of central sleep apnea and ataxic breathing. Journal of Clinical Sleep Medicine. 2007;**03**:455-461. DOI: 10.5664/jcsm.26908

[154] Elbassiony A, Khedr EM, Hegazy A, Ragab OA, Al-Shami H, Soliman RK, et al. The frequency and impact of tramadol addiction on acute aneurysmal subarachnoid hemorrhage: Cross-sectional multicenter study. Egyptian Journal of Neurology, Psychiatry and Neurosurgery. 2023;**59**:97. DOI: 10.1186/s41983-023-00703-w

[155] Baldo BA, Rose MA. Mechanisms of opioid-induced respiratory depression. Archives of Toxicology. 2022;**96**:2247-2260. DOI: 10.1007/s00204-022-03300-7

[156] Montandon G. The pathophysiology of opioid-induced respiratory depression2022. pp. 339-355. DOI: 10.1016/B978-0-323-91534-2.00003-5

[157] Guan Q, Men S, Juurlink DN, Bronskill SE, Wunsch H, Gomes T. Opioid initiation and the Hazard of falls or fractures among older adults with varying levels of central nervous system depressant burden. Drugs & Aging. 2022;**39**:729-738. DOI: 10.1007/s40266-022-00970-x

[158] Mousa RF, Smesam HN, Qazmooz HA, Al-Hakeim HK,

Maes M. A pathway phenotype linking metabolic, immune, oxidative, and opioid pathways with comorbid depression, atherosclerosis, and unstable angina. CNS Spectrums. 2022;**27**:676-690. DOI: 10.1017/S1092852921000432

[159] Toska E, Mayrovitz HN. Opioid impacts on cardiovascular health. Cureus. 2023:e46224. DOI: 10.7759/cureus.46224

[160] Liang L, Chen J, Zhang C, Luo B, Zhou T, Wang X, et al. Association of Lipoprotein-associated phospholipase A2 with carotid intima-media thickness in acute cerebral infarction patients. Angiology. 2024:1842-1855. DOI: 10.1177/00033197241233774

[161] Yigit E, Yasar S, Can M, Bayraktar Z. Gout and erectile dysfunction: Increased carotid intima-media thickness is independently associated with greater likelihood for erectile dysfunction. Archives of Rheumatology. 2024;**39**:393-403. DOI: 10.46497/ArchRheumatol.2024.10486

[162] Lin N, Mandel D, Chuck CC, Kalagara R, Doelfel SR, Zhou H, et al. Risk factors for opioid utilization in patients with intracerebral hemorrhage. Neurocritical Care. 2022;**36**:964-973. DOI: 10.1007/s12028-021-01404-z

[163] Mahta A, Anderson MN, Azher AI, Mahmoud LN, Dakay K, Abdulrazeq H, et al. Short- and long-term opioid use in survivors of subarachnoid hemorrhage. Clinical Neurology and Neurosurgery. 2021;**207**:106770. DOI: 10.1016/j.clineuro.2021.106770

[164] Behroozi Z, Jafarpour M, Razmgir M, Saffarpour S, Azizi H, Kheirandish A, et al. The effect of gabapentin and pregabalin administration on memory in clinical and preclinical studies: A meta-analysis and systematic review. BMC Psychiatry. 2023;**23**:262. DOI: 10.1186/s12888-023-04696-x

[165] Almutairi S, Sivadas A, Kwakowsky A. The effect of oral GABA on the nervous system: Potential for therapeutic intervention. Nutraceuticals. 2024;**4**:241-259. DOI: 10.3390/nutraceuticals4020015

[166] Slocum GW, Schult RF, Gorodetsky RM, Wiegand TJ, Kamali M, Acquisto NM. Pregabalin and paradoxical reaction of seizures in a large overdose. Toxicology Communications. 2018;**2**:19-20. DOI: 10.1080/24734306.2018.1458465

[167] Testai FD, Gorelick PB, Aparicio HJ, Filbey FM, Gonzalez R, Gottesman RF, et al. Use of marijuana: Effect on brain health: A scientific statement from the American Heart Association. Stroke. 2022;**53**(4):e176-e187. DOI: 10.1161/STR.0000000000000396

[168] Gueyraud G, Guidolin B, Olivot J, Lerebours F, Barbieux-Guillot M, Larrue V, et al. Stroke phenotype in cannabis users among young adults with ischemic stroke. European Journal of Neurology. 2023;**30**:1891-1898. DOI: 10.1111/ene.15799

[169] Swetlik C, Migdady I, Hasan LZ, Buletko AB, Price C, Cho S-M. Cannabis use and stroke: Does a risk exist? Journal of Addiction Medicine. 2022;**16**:208-215. DOI: 10.1097/ADM.0000000000000870

[170] Short K, Emsley HCA. Illicit drugs and reversible cerebral vasoconstriction syndrome. The Neurohospitalist. 2021;**11**:40-44. DOI: 10.1177/1941874420953051

[171] Bliss L, McGowan B, Rahman A. A rare pediatric case of marijuana-induced

reversible cerebral vasoconstriction syndrome. Pediatric Neurology. 2021;**120**:33-35. DOI: 10.1016/j.pediatrneurol.2021.03.008

[172] Moustafa B, Testai FD. Cerebrovascular complications associated with marijuana use. Current Neurology and Neuroscience Reports. 2021;**21**:25. DOI: 10.1007/s11910-021-01113-2

[173] Da Cunha ND, Petriz B, Da Cunha OS, Vieira DCL, Funghetto SS, Silva AO, et al. Effects of blood flow restriction exercise on hemostasis: A systematic review of randomized and non-randomized trials. International Journal of General Medicine. 2019;**12**:91-100. DOI: 10.2147/IJGM.S194883

[174] Hooper P, Jutai JW, Strong G, Russell-Minda E. Age-related macular degeneration and low-vision rehabilitation: A systematic review. Canadian Journal of Ophthalmology. 2008;**43**:180-187. DOI: 10.3129/I08-001